HEALTH
CARE
DEFINED

A Glossary of
Current Terms

HEALTH CARE DEFINED

A Glossary of
Current Terms

Bruce Goldfarb

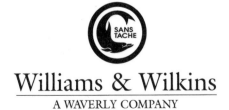

Williams & Wilkins

A WAVERLY COMPANY

BALTIMORE • PHILADELPHIA • LONDON • PARIS • BANGKOK
BUENOS AIRES • HONG KONG • MUNICH • SYDNEY • TOKYO • WROCLAW

Editor: Elizabeth Randolph
Managing Editor: Maureen Barlow Pugh
Production Coordinator: Raymond E. Reter
Designer: Wilma Rosenberger
Typesetter: Graphic Sciences Corporation, Cedar Rapids, Iowa
Printer & Binder: Vicks Lithograph & Printing Corporation, Yorkville, New York

351 West Camden Street
Baltimore, Maryland 21201-2436 USA

Rose Tree Corporate Center
1400 North Providence Road
Building II, Suite 5025
Media, Pennsylvania 19063-2043 USA

Printed in the United States of America

Library of Congress Cataloging-in-Publication Data

Goldfarb, Bruce.
    Health care defined : a glossary of current terms / Bruce
Goldfarb.
        p.   cm.
    ISBN 0-683-03615-7
    1. Medical care—Dictionaries.   I. Title.
RA423.G65   1996
362.1'03—dc20   96-31716
                                                                                    CIP

The publishers have made every effort to trace the copyright holders for borrowed material. If they have inadvertently overlooked any, they will be pleased to make the necessary arrangements at the first opportunity.

To purchase additional copies of this book, call our customer service department at **(800) 638-0672** or fax orders to **(800) 447-8438.** For other book services, including chapter reprints and large quantity sales, ask for the Special Sales department.

Canadian customers should call **(800) 268-4178,** or fax **(905) 470-6780.** For all other calls originating outside of the United States, please call **(410) 528-4223** or fax us at **(410) 528-8550.**

Visit Williams & Wilkins on the Internet: **http://www.wwilkins.com** or contact our customer service department at **custserv@wwilkins.com.** Williams & Wilkins customer service representatives are available from 8:30 am to 6:00 pm, EST, Monday through Friday, for telephone access.

                                                                    96 97 98 99 00
                                                            1 2 3 4 5 6 7 8 9 10

For Helane and George

PREFACE

The US health care system is undergoing dramatic develop-
ments that are fundamentally changing the relationships between
patients, the providers of health care services, and those who pay
for it. Medicine in years past was a simple endeavor; patients were
treated by doctors, sometimes put in the hospital, and an insurance
company or other responsible party paid the bills.

Spiraling medical costs led to managed care — strategies to control costs while improving the quality of health care delivery. New
layers of administration have emerged to ensure that health care is
appropriate and cost effective. More recently, the emphasis has
turned to measuring the outcomes of medical care and continually
improving the quality of health care services.

The health care system brings together professionals in widely
divergent disciplines — including clinical medicine, administration, social services and finance — each with its own unique language. Along with the new paradigm of health care has come a
confusing alphabet soup of acronyms and jargon.

The goal of *Health Care Defined* was to produce a concise yet
comprehensive guide to terminology currently used in the delivery
of health care. It is intended to be a convenient and quick reference
that defines the most commonly used terms. One hopes that this
reference can contribute to greater understanding, and enhance
the ability of different disciplines to work collaboratively as the
health care system continues to evolve in the future.

Many people contributed invaluable assistance in the course of
this project. Elizabeth Randolph is as amiable an editor as one can
wish for. Maureen Barlow Pugh kindly kept me on task and gave
shape to the glossary's final form. Dave Horne, a top-notch pro-
grammer who designed the software, invariably responded quickly
to my numerous crises. I appreciate the thoughtful comments of
Susan Alt, Barb Hamilton, Robert Hogan, MD, Rick Urbanski, and
John Walsh. Most of all, I am grateful for the love and support of
my wife, Nancy, and my sons, Max and Phillip.

Bruce Goldfarb

PUBLISHER'S PREFACE

Health Care Defined: A Glossary of Current Terms is an up-to-date and accessible reference that defines terms commonly used in the health care industry. It was designed specifically to help those involved in health care services delivery, insurance, and law.

Users of *Health Care Defined* will find it to be a convenient, authoritative guide to the spelling and meaning of the commonly used words and phrases, jargon, abbreviations and acronyms used in managed care, insurance and reimbursement, health care administration, ambulatory care management, health care law and finance, quality improvement, health information systems management, integrated systems, workers' compensation, rehabilitation, medical records and transcription, medical social work, allied health, and clinical medicine.

By pulling together terms of interest to the many segments of health care in one place, we hope that *Health Care Defined* will facilitate communication among professionals involved in the delivery or administration of health care services.

We at Williams & Wilkins strive to provide students, practitioners, and educators with the most up-to-date and accurate medical language references available. Your use of this glosssary will prompt new editions, published as often as needed. We welcome your suggestions for improvements, changes, corrections, and additions — whatever will make this reference product more useful to you.

CONTENTS

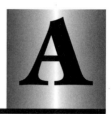

A
1. allergy
2. anterior
3. assessment

AA
1. Alcoholics Anonymous
2. anesthesiologist's assistant

AAACN
American Academy of Ambulatory Care Nursing

AAAHC
Accreditation Association for Ambulatory Health Care

AAAI
American Academy of Allergy and Immunology

AABB
American Association of Blood Banks

AABD
Aid to the Aged, Blind and Disabled

AACC
American Association for Continuity of Care

AAD
American Academy of Dermatology

AAFP
American Academy of Family Physicians

AAHC
American Association of Healthcare Consultants

AAHP
American Association of Health Plans

AAMCN
American Association of Managed Care Nurses

AAMT
American Association for Medical Transcription

AAN
American Academy of Neurology

AANP
American Academy of Nurse Practitioners

AAO
1. American Academy of Ophthalmology
2. American Academy of Osteopathy

AAOS
American Academy of Orthopedic Surgeons

AAP
1. American Academy of Pediatrics
2. American Accreditation Program

AAPCC
adjusted average per capita cost

AAPE
American Association of Physician Executives

AAPHO
American Association of Physician-Hospital Organizations

AAPMR
American Academy of Physical Medicine and Rehabilitation

AAPPO
American Association of Preferred Provider Organizations

AB
1. abortion
2. aid to the blind

abandonment
1. The act of leaving an ill or injured patient without another person to take responsibility for providing care.
2. The intentional desertion of a child.
3. The termination of the patient-provider relationship without properly informing the patient and allowing sufficient time, notice or opportunity to obtain care by another provider.

ABG
arterial blood gas

ABIM
American Board of Internal Medicine

ABMS
American Board of Medical Specialties

abortion
The termination of a pregnancy before the fetus is viable, i.e., able to survive outside of the womb. Abortions can occur spontaneously and also result from treatment intended to terminate the pregnancy.
SEE ALSO: still birth

ABPM
American Board of Preventive Medicine

ABS
abdominal surgery

abstinence
Refraining from use, e.g., of alcohol or sex.

abstract
A summary that gives an overview of a subject or document.

abuse
1. Improper or wrong use, e.g., substance abuse.
2. The inappropriate use of a resource, such as a service or program.
3. The mistreatment or harm of another person.

abuse, child
SEE: child abuse

abuse, elder
> *SEE:* elder abuse

abuse, spousal
> *SEE:* spousal abuse

abuse, system
> *SEE:* system abuse

ac
> before meals

ACA
> American Chiropractic Association

ACC
> Ambulatory Care Center

accelerated death benefit
> Money paid prior to death to a terminally ill person covered by a
> life insurance policy.
> > *SYN:* viatical settlement
> > viatication

acceptability
> The level of satisfaction patients report about health care services.

access
> The ability of clients to gain entry and use a health care facility or
> service. Barriers to access may be physical, economic, or social.

accession number
> In medical records, a unique sequential number assigned to or-
> ders as they are submitted.

accident
> An unintentional, unforseen, and unexpected event.
> > *SEE ALSO:* injury
> > trauma

accident and health insurance
> A contract between an individual and a company in which the
> insurer agrees to pay medical and hospital expenses in the event
> of disease or trauma, or death benefits in the event of death, in
> return of payment of premiums.

accidental bodily harm
An insurance term for unintentional physical injury.

accidental death and dismemberment (AD&D)
Coverage that pays an amount of money in the event an insured person dies or is dismembered as a result of an accident.

accidental death benefit
A benefit paid to the estate of an insured person in addition to the face value of a life insurance policy in the event the insured dies as a result of an accident.
Syn: double indemnity

accidental injury
See: unintentional injury

accountable health partnership
See: accountable health plan

accountable health plan (AHP)
A proposed organization that contracts with employer groups, cooperatives, or alliances for health care services rendered at a fixed annual rate. The organization would have provider network and health insurance components and be required to meet national health benefit standards.
Syn: accountable health partnership
approved health plan

accounting, accrual
See: accrual accounting

accounting, cash
See: cash accounting

accounts receivable (AR)
Billed charges as yet unpaid by the patient, insurer, or other payer.

accounts receivable ratio (ARR)
The number of months of revenue in accounts receivable; a measurement of the duration until payment is collected for services rendered.

ACCP
American College of Chest Physicians

accreditation
Certification by an independent nonprofit organization that a health care provider, facility, service, or program meets or exceeds specific minimum standards.

accrediting organization
An independent, nonprofit group that grants accreditation.

accrete
To enroll a Medicare recipient in a health plan.

accrual
1. A gain of something.
2. A method of accounting in which costs and revenues are calculated over a period of time regardless of whether money is exchanged during that time.
3. An amount of money designated for the expenses of a health benefit plan.
   SEE ALSO: cash accounting

accrual accounting
A bookkeeping method that records costs and revenues as they occur. In managed care, costs for a group of persons are estimated for a period of time, such as one month. A claims reserve employed to cover expenses generated during the time period.
   SEE ALSO: cash accounting
         claims reserve

accruals
Short-term debts that continually occur, such as wages and taxes.

accrued expenses
Funds consumed by a hospital or health care entity, in the course of normal operations, that have not yet been billed by or paid to the vendor.

accumulation
1. A provision in some health insurance policies that increases the level of benefits as an incentive for continued renewal.
2. The total number of services utilized by a patient under a benefit plan that limits costs or office visits.

accumulation period
Time interval in which an insured's medical expenses accumulate for consideration in deductible requirements, such as a calendar year.

ACE
angiotensin-converting enzyme

ACEP
American College of Emergency Physicians

ACHA
American College of Healthcare Executives

acid test ratio
A measure of financial liquidity determined by dividing current assets by current liabilities.

ACLA
American Clinical Laboratory Association

ACLS
advanced cardiac life support

ACMQ
American College of Medical Quality

ACOG
American College of Obstetricians and Gynecologists

ACP
American College of Physicians

acquisition
The purchase of the assets or majority voting interest of a corporation, through the exchange of cash, assets or other compensation.

acquisition cost
An insurance company's costs associated with issuing a policy, such as home-office expenses and agent commissions.

acquisition, stock
SEE: stock acquisition

ACR
1. adjusted community rating
2. American College of Rheumatology

ACS
1. American Cancer Society
2. American College of Surgeons

ACTH
adrenocorticotrophic hormone

activities of daily living (ADL)
Actions typically associated with normal daily life, such as washing, dressing, and eating. A patient's ADL abilities are evaluated to assess the continuing needs for care.

actuarial analysis
The statistical analysis of loss exposures, historical loss experience, and related factors for the purpose of estimating financial obligations and the determination of health insurance premiums.

actuarial assumptions
Economic forecasts, environmental factors, and historical loss analysis factors considered by an actuary in determining risks, revenues, and costs. Examples of actuarial assumptions include the demographic mix of enrollees and the utilization rates of health care services.

actuarial cost model
An analysis of the probability and magnitude, or cost, of an event.

actuary
A person trained in statistics and accounting who uses the calculation of probability to determine the rate of policy premiums, the amount of reserves, and dividends.

acupressure
A form of alternative medicine similar to acupuncture, using massage rather than needles.

acupuncture
A system of alternative medicine featuring the use of thin needles that are believed to redirect energy when placed along meridians of the body. Sometimes used to manage chronic conditions, such as pain and addictions.

acute
Having a rapid and severe onset.
SEE ALSO: chronic

acute care
Short-term care for patients with acute illness or injury.
SEE ALSO: chronic care
            hospitalization
            long-term care

acute episode
An incident in which a chronic illness becomes markedly severe, requiring more intensive treatment for a period of time.

acute illness
A single episode of a disease or other condition marked by a rapid and severe onset. Usually, the patient recovers within a short duration to his or her previous level of function.
SEE ALSO: chronic illness

AD
1. Associate Degree
2. right ear

ADA
1. American Dental Association
2. Americans with Disabilities Act

adaptation
The ability to meet the demands of the environment.

adaptive technology
Devices to compensate for physical limitations, such as low-vision glasses, motorized wheelchairs, and speech-synthesis machines.

ADC
1. Aid to Families with Dependent Children
2. average daily census

ADD
attention deficit disorder

AD&D
accidental death and dismemberment

addict
A person with an uncontrollable habit, such as the use of drugs.

addiction
The habitual abuse of a drug, the absence of which causes physical or psychological symptoms of withdrawal.
    SEE ALSO: drug abuse

ADF
administrative determination of fault

ADFS
alternative delivery and financing system

ADGC
average daily gross charges

ADGR
average daily gross revenue

adhesion
1. A legal principle in which ambiguous or unclear wording in an insurance agreement is interpreted against the insurer and in favor of the insured.
2. The physical attraction between two unlike molecules.
3. The union of two tissue surfaces, such as the two sides of a wound.

ADI
acceptable daily intake

adjudication
The processing of health care claims according to the terms of a benefit contract.

adjusted average per capita cost (AAPCC)
An estimate used by the Health Care Financing Administration to determine health care costs for Medicare recipients under a fee-for-service system, with adjustments for age and gender.

adjusted community rating
The use of group-specific demographics, such as age, in community rating.
SEE ALSO: community rating

adjuster
A person employed by an insurance company who determines the dollar amount of a claim or debt.
SYN: health insurance adjuster

adjustment
The settling of the amount the insured is entitled to receive under an insurance policy.

adjustment, administrative
SEE: administrative adjustment

adjustment, area wage
SEE: area wage adjustment

adjustment, risk
SEE: risk adjustment

adjustments
Credits to patient account balances because of refunds, professional courtesy, contractual obligations, bad debt, or some other reason.

adjustment, volume
SEE: volume adjustment

ADL
1. activities of daily living
2. adolescent medicine

ad lib.
as desired

administer
To direct or manage an organization, service, or program.

administration
1. The delivery of a dose of medication or treatment to a patient.
2. The management, supervision, planning, and execution activities of an organization that help accomplish its goals and objectives.

administrative
Related to general management activities other than the direct provision of care to patients.

administrative adjustment
An accounting method to show that services were provided but not billed to patients because the cost of billing and collection would exceed the actual charges.

administrative agent
SEE: third-party administrator

administrative costs
Expenses associated with the operation of a health benefit plan, such as agents' commissions, premium collection, claims processing, marketing, utilization review, and quality assurance.

administrative determination of fault (ADF)
A form of alternative dispute resolution in which an independent agency is designated to adjudicate medical malpractice cases. Claimants may be compensated from a special fund established for this purpose.
SEE ALSO: alternative dispute resolution

administrative load
The portion of health care costs attributable to administration and marketing.
SYN: retention

administrative loading
The amount of money in a premium added to the actuarial costs of health services to cover overhead expenses, such as marketing, administration, and profit.

administrative services contract
SEE: administrative services only

administrative services only (ASO)
A contractual arrangement between a self-insured group and an insurance company for administration and stop-loss coverage.
SYN: administrative services contract
SEE ALSO: self-insurance

administrator
A chief executive officer or other executive who carries out the mission, goals, objectives, and other functions of a health care organization.

administrator, qualified
SEE: qualified administrator

administrator, third-party
SEE: third-party administrator

admission and discharge dates
The day, month, and year that a patient is admitted and discharged from a medical or mental health facility.

admission certification
A medical review to assess the necessity of a patient's admission to a hospital or other inpatient facility.
SEE ALSO: utilization review

admission date
The calendar date on which a patient is formally accepted into a health care facility or program.

admission diagnosis
A presumptive diagnosis made at the time of a patient's admission to a hospital. The diagnosis may change depending on laboratory tests, diagnostic procedures, and physical examination of the patient.

SYN: admitting diagnosis
provisional diagnosis
tentative diagnosis

admission, elective
SEE: elective admission

admission, emergency
SEE: emergency admission

admission, newborn
SEE: newborn admission

admission notification
A communication from a hospital or other health facility to the insurer or payer to inform of a patient's admission status and determine eligibility for health benefit coverage.

admission pattern monitoring
SEE: APM

admissions
The number of patients in an inpatient medical facility or extended care facility during a specified time period.
SYN: admits

admission, urgent
SEE: urgent admission

admit rate
The volume of admissions to a hospital during a specified time period. Usually expressed as an annual rate per 1,000 persons.

admits
SEE: admissions

admitting diagnosis
SEE: admission diagnosis

admitting privileges
An arrangement between a physician and a hospital allowing the admission of patients and use of the hospital's staff and facilities.

ADR
alternative dispute resolution

ADS
alternative delivery system

adult day care
A program providing health, psychological, social, and other supportive services to help elderly or infirm adults remain in the home.

adult foster care
SEE: assisted-living facility

adults-only housing
SEE: seniors' apartments

adults, vulnerable
SEE: vulnerable adults

advance directive
A legal document prepared by a person to express wishes regarding medical intervention in the event he or she becomes incapacitated and unable to make decisions.
SEE ALSO: living will

advanced emergency medical technician
SEE: paramedic

advanced practice nurse
SEE: APN

adverse patient outcome
1. A biological or psychological decremental change in health status.
2. Death.
SYN: mortality

adverse selection
The disproportionate enrollment in a pre-paid health plan of persons with greater-than-average need for health care services.

advocacy
Activities and efforts directed at promoting the interests of an individual or group.

aerobic exercise
Sustained physical activity that maintains a high heart rate and respiratory rate.
SYN: aerobics

aerobics
SEE: aerobic exercise

aeromedical service
The use of fixed-wing aircraft or helicopter, staffed with trained professionals, to transport patients to a hospital or transfer between facilities.
SYN: air evac

AFACAL
Associate Fellow of the American College of Allergists

AFDC
Aid to Families with Dependent Children

afebrile
Without fever.

affected person
An individual residing within the geographic area served by a rate increase or certificate of need.

affiliation
An agreement among providers, such as a physician and a hospital, with explicitly defined roles and relationships. May range from informal joint marketing agreements to formalized exclusive contracts or joint ownership and control.

affiliation, hospital
SEE: hospital affiliation

AFHHA
American Federation of Home Health Agencies

AFIP
Armed Forces Institute of Pathology

AFS
alternative financing system

aftercare
Continued follow-up contact with patients after the acute phase of treatment to monitor progress and maximize the level of recovery.
SEE ALSO: discharge planning

after-hours care
The delivery of health services outside of a provider or outpatient facility's usual business hours. May include telephone referral to another provider, an emergency department, or to another facility.

against medical advice (AMA)
The discharge status of a patient who leaves the hospital contrary to the opinion of the treating physician and/or staff. Typically, the patient will be asked to sign a document relieving providers of liability.
SEE ALSO: discharge status

age limits
1. Limitations in health benefits when a beneficiary reaches a specified age.
2. Specified maximum and minimum ages beyond which an insurance company will not issue or renew a policy for coverage.

agency
1. A governmental organization designated by law as responsible for specific administrative duties, such as the regulation of goods and services.
2. A private company that provides a health care service, i.e., a home health agency.

agency, home health
SEE: home health agency

age-sex rates
Actuarial tables used to calculate the premiums for a group of individuals.
SYN: table rates

age-sex rating (ASR)
A method of calculating capitated payments to providers based on the age and gender of patients.
SYN: table rating

aggregate amount
The maximum amount for which a beneficiary is covered for any single event.

aggregate, lifetime
SEE: lifetime aggregate

aging analysis
The measurement of accounts receivable by grouping unpaid patient accounts into categories based on the duration since services were rendered, such as 0–30 days, 31–60 days and so on.

AGPA
American Group Practice Association

agreement, confidentiality
SEE: confidentiality agreement

agreement, reserve reduction
SEE: reserve reduction agreement

agreement, third-party
SEE: third-party agreement

AHA
1. American Heart Association
2. American Hospital Association

AHCA
American Health Care Association

AHCPR
Agency for Health Care Policy and Research

AHEC
area health education center

AHIMA
American Health Information Management Association

AHP
1. accountable health partnership
2. accountable health plan
3. approved health plan

AI
1. allergy and immunology
2. artificial intelligence

AID
artificial insemination by donor

AIDS
Acquired immunodeficiency syndrome. A disease caused by the human immunodeficiency virus (HIV) characterized by opportunistic infections and malignancies.

AIH
artificial insemination by husband

AIP
annual implementation plan

air evac
SEE: aeromedical service

alb
albumin

algorithm, clinical
SEE: treatment protocol

algorithm, treatment
SEE: treatment protocol

allergist
A physician who specializes in the diagnosis and treatment of allergies.

allergy and immunology
The study of contagious disease and allergies.

alliance
1. A formalized collaborative arrangement among companies, providers or institutions, created to further common goals.
2. An entity that purchases health insurance.
3. An organization of employers that pool resources for the purposes of purchasing health care goods and services.

allied health personnel
All non-physician health care staff involved in patient care, including physician's assistants, nurses, aides, assistants, technicians, and therapists.
SYN: allied health professionals

allied health professionals
SEE: allied health personnel

allocated benefits
Health benefits for which the maximum payable amount for specific goods or services is itemized in the contract.

allocation of overhead
The assignment of overhead expenses to specific patient care areas, based on such factors as physical space, staffing size or manpower hours.

allocation of risk
A mechanism by which uninsurable small employers are equitably assigned among insurers.

allograft
The surgical transplantation of tissue donated by a person other than the patient.
SEE ALSO: homograft

allopathy
A medical approach in which the treatment is the opposite of the condition which the patient suffers.
SEE ALSO: homeopathy

allowable charges
Medical goods or services that are eligible for reimbursement under a health benefit plan.
SYN: allowables

allowables
SEE: allowable charges

allowance, charity
SEE: charity allowance

allowed amount
The maximum dollar amount paid for a medical procedure according to guidelines used by an insurer or managed care company.
SYN: maximum allowable

all-payer system
A proposal in which uniform prices would be imposed on medical services regardless of the payer, so that all would pay the same price. Eliminates cost-shifting to those who are better able to pay.
SEE ALSO: cost-shifting
third-party payer

ALOS
average length of stay

ALS
1. advanced life support
2. amyotrophic lateral sclerosis

alternate benefit
A provision of some health plan contracts that allows a third-party payer to base benefits on a less expensive alternate procedure. Given two procedures of equal efficacy and safety, the payer may opt to cover only the cost of the less expensive one.

alternate treatment, least expensive
SEE: least expensive alternative treatment

alternative delivery and financing system (ADFS)
A system of delivering and financing health services that is an alternative to traditional fee-for-service, e.g., a health maintenance organization.
SEE ALSO: fee-for-service
health maintenance organization

alternative delivery mode
>   *SEE:* alternative delivery system

alternative delivery system (ADS)
1. An arrangement of providers other than solo practice and traditional small groups, i.e., health maintenance organization (HMO), preferred provider organization (PPO), independent practice association (IPA), or exclusive provider organization (EPO).
2. Health services outside of traditional hospital care, such as home health care and ambulatory care.
>   *SYN:* alternative delivery mode

alternative dispute resolution (ADR)
Arrangements to resolve malpractice claims other than litigation, such as arbitration or administrative determination of fault (ADF).
>   *SEE ALSO:* administrative determination of fault
>   arbitration

alternative financing system (AFS)
A system for financing health care services that is an alternative to fee-for-service, such as capitation.

alternative health care
>   *SEE:* alternative medicine

alternative medicine
Health remedies that are not within mainstream medicine.
>   *SYN:* alternative health care

a.m.
before noon

AM
aerospace medicine

AMA
1. against medical advice
2. American Medical Association

ambulatory care
Health care services that are provided on an outpatient basis, without admission for an overnight stay in a hospital.
SYN: outpatient care

ambulatory care facility
A facility, either based at a hospital or free-standing, that provides care on an outpatient basis, without the need for an overnight stay in a hospital. May provide diagnostic services, preventive care, emergency medicine, minor surgery or other services.
SYN: clinic
day surgery
outpatient facility

ambulatory care system
A formalized organization centered around outpatient health services—physicians, nurses, ancillary services, and access to hospital-based services.

ambulatory patient group
SEE: APG

ambulatory surgery
The performance of surgical procedures and related care to outpatients, who are not admitted for an overnight stay in a hospital and are usually discharged within a few hours of surgery.
SYN: 23-hour surgery
come-and-go surgery
day surgery
one-day surgery
outpatient surgery
short-stay surgery

ambulatory surgery categories (ASC)
A system for classifying ambulatory surgery patients into meaningful groups.
SEE ALSO: diagnosis-related groups
major diagnostic categories

ambulatory visit group (AVG)
A system of classifying ambulatory care patients into related diagnoses for the purposes of applying a predetermined rate of reimbursement.
SEE ALSO: diagnosis related group

AMCP
Academy of Managed Care Pharmacy

AMCRA
American Managed Care and Review Association
SEE: American Association of Health Plans

AMCS
automated medical coding system.

AMI
acute myocardial infarction

amount, aggregate
SEE: aggregate amount

amount, approved
SEE: approved amount

AMPRA
American Medical Peer Review Association

amt
amount

AN
anesthesiology

ANA
American Nurses Association

analysis, actuarial
SEE: actuarial analysis

analysis, aging
SEE: aging analysis

analysis, retrospective
SEE: retrospective review

analysis, variance
    SEE: variance analysis

anatomy
    1. Dissection.
    2. Study of the structures of an organism.

anatomy, gross
    SEE: gross anatomy

anatomy, microscopic
    SEE: microscopic anatomy

ancillary charges
    Hospital charges in addition to daily room and board, which may include medications, diagnostic testing, operating room costs, and charges for patient care supplies.

ancillary services
    Hospital services other than nursing care and "room and board," e.g. laboratories, diagnostic and radiological services, pharmacy, physical therapy, rehabilitation and home health care.
    SYN: auxiliary services
         miscellaneous services

anesthesia
    1. A general term for the specialty of anesthesiology.
    2. The administration of drugs or gasses to induce a state marked by the absence of sensation, usually produced for the purposes of a pain-free surgical procedure.

anesthesiologist
    A physician who specializes in the administration of anesthesia, the control of pain and related areas.
    SYN: gas passer
    SEE ALSO: anesthesiology

anesthesiology
    The medical specialty concerned with anesthesia, resuscitation, critical care medicine and control of pain.

anesthetic
1. Characterized by a loss of sensation.
2. Medications used to depress the function of the nervous system.

anesthetist
A person who administers an anesthetic. May be a physician, nurse or technician.
SEE ALSO: anesthesiology

anesthetist, nurse
SEE: nurse anesthetist

angiography
The creation of a radiographic image of a blood vessel injected with a radiopaque dye.

anniversary
The date denoting the beginning of a subscriber group's benefit year.
SYN: anniversary date

anniversary date
SEE: anniversary

ANS
autonomic nervous system

anti-dumping law
Federal regulations prohibiting the transfer or discharge of patients because of the inability to pay for care.
SEE ALSO: Consolidated Omnibus Budget Reconciliation Act of 1985
patient dumping

anti-kickback laws
Legal restrictions on payments and other incentives that are unfair business practices.
SEE ALSO: antitrust

antipruritic
A drug that relieves itching.

antiseptic
A substance that inhibits the growth of microorganisms.

antitrust
Regulation of an industry to prevent unfair business practices, such as restraint of trade and elimination of competition.

any willing provider (AWP)
State law prohibiting discrimination against health care providers; requires managed care networks to accept any provider willing to accept the payor's terms.
SYN: "freedom of choice" law
SEE ALSO: closed panel
"patient protection" law
preferred provider

AOB
assignment of benefits

AOHA
American Osteopathic Healthcare Association

AP
1. accounts payable
2. anterior-posterior

A&P
1. anatomy and physiology
2. anterior and posterior

APA
1. American Pharmaceutical Association
2. American Psychiatric Association
3. American Psychological Association

APG
ambulatory patient group

APHA
American Public Health Association

APM
admission pattern monitoring

APMA
American Podiatric Medicine Association

APN
advanced practice nurse

APO
adverse patient outcome

appropriate certifying agency
SEE: appropriate certifying authority

appropriate certifying authority
A state organization that certifies qualified health plans, generally under the insurance commission or the department of health, or their equivalents.

SYN: appropriate certifying agency

appropriateness
The determination whether a given course of treatment is correct based on the nature of the patient's condition and the standards of medical care.

approved amount
An amount of money determined by a Medicare carrier as reasonable and fair reimbursement for health care services.

approved health plan
SEE: accountable health plan

approved research trial
A clinical research protocol sanctioned by the Secretary of Health and Human Services, the National Institutes of Health, the Food and Drug Administration, the Department of Veterans Affairs, or a qualified non-governmental research institution.

APR
average payment rate

APS
attending physician statement

APTD
aid to the permanently and totally disabled

aq
water

AQL
acceptable quality level

AR
accounts receivable

ARA
American Rehabilitation Association

arbitration
Any means of resolving disputes or disagreements by having a determination made by a disinterested third party, either an individual or panel. Arbitration is an administrative rather than judicial process.

arbitration, binding
SEE: binding arbitration

ARC
AIDS-related complex

area, service
SEE: service area

area wage adjustment
In a prospective payment system, a factor used in formulating payments that accounts for geographic differences in wages.

aromatherapy
A form of alternative medicine in which essential oils are inhaled or absorbed by the skin.

ARR
accounts receivable ratio

arrest, cardiac
SEE: cardiac arrest

ART
accredited record technician

art therapy
Use of art for therapeutic purposes.

AS
left ear

ASC
1. administrative services contract
2. ambulatory surgery categories
3. ambulatory surgical center

ASD
atrial septal defect

ASHD
atherosclerotic heart disease

ASHRM
American Society for Healthcare Risk Management

ASO
administrative services only

ASPRS
American Society of Plastic and Reconstructive Surgery

ASR
1. age-sex rates
2. age-sex rating

assay
An analysis to determine the presence of a substance in a sample.
    SYN: test

assessment
An organized process for gathering relevant clinical information about the health status of a patient.

assignment
The transfer of insurance benefits from the beneficiary directly to another party, often to the provider. The provider may accept assignment, and responsibility for collection, or require payment from the beneficiary.
    SEE ALSO: balance billing
                mandatory assignment

assignment, mandatory
> *SEE:* mandatory assignment

assignment of benefits
> Permission granted by the insured for benefit to be paid directly to health care providers.

assisted-living facility
> A housing arrangement that provides assistance with activities of daily living, such as bathing or cooking, but not skilled nursing services.
> *SYN:* adult foster care

association, independent practice
> *SEE:* independent practice association

assumptions, actuarial
> *SEE:* actuarial assumptions

ATA
> American Thoracic Association

ATP
> anatomic pathology

at risk
> The liability to which an entity is exposed when it is paid a fixed amount for the provision of specific health care services. If the costs of those services exceeds the amount paid, the company or provider loses money.

at-risk
> A population with greater-than-average likelihood of acquiring a specific illness or injury.

attained age
> An individual's age at his or her last birthday.

attending physician
> 1. A medical doctor who is primarily responsible for the care of a patient during hospitalization.
> 2. A physician with a medical practice affiliated with a hospital.

attending physician statement (APS)
A report completed by a physician documenting the current and past health history of an applicant or claimant.

attorney-client privilege
Legal principles protecting the confidentiality of communication between an attorney and the client being represented.

attrition rate
The percentage of total HMO membership that disenroll within a defined time period, usually a month.
SYN: fall-out rate

AU
both ears

AUA
American Urological Association

audit
The determination of the accuracy of records and documents. Audits are performed to verify information and the delivery of services and to check whether charges are accurate and reasonable.

audit, interdisciplinary
SEE: interdisciplinary audit

audit study
The review and evaluation of health care services.

audit study sample
A representative group of patients or services reviewed for an audit study.

audit study subject
A category chosen for evaluation of health care services, such as a diagnostic group or surgical procedure.

authorization
Approval given by a managed care company for hospitalization or referral to a medical specialist.

authorization, written
>*SEE:* written authorization

automated clinical analyzer
Computerized clinical laboratory equipment that performs chemical tests on blood and body fluids.

auxiliary procedure
A procedure that is not the primary reason for the patient encounter, consuming a small portion of the time and resources spent with the patient.

auxiliary services
>*SEE:* ancillary services

auxiliary test
A test ordered by the primary physician to assist in the diagnosis and treatment of the patient, but is not definitive or of major importance.

AV
atrioventricular

availability
The presence, absence, or capacity of a health service or program in a community.

average census
>*SEE:* average daily census

average daily census (ADC)
The mean or median number of patients each day in a health care facility.
>*SYN:* average census
>average daily number of inpatients

average daily gross charges (ADGC)
The average billed charges for each day during a period of time.

average daily gross revenue (ADGR)
The average revenue for each day during a period of time.

average daily number of inpatients
>*SEE:* average daily census

average duration of hospitalization
The mean or median length of stay of patients in a health care facility
SYN: average duration of stay
SEE ALSO: average length of stay

average duration of stay
SEE: average duration of hospitalization

average length of stay (ALOS)
The average duration of inpatient stays, expressed in days.

average stay
SEE: average duration of hospitalization

AVG
ambulatory visit group

AWP
1. any willing provider
2. average wholesale price

ayurveda
A form of alternative medicine originating in India involving special diets, cleansing, and meditation.
SYN: ayurvedic medicine

ayurvedic medicine
SEE: ayurveda

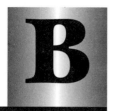

baby, boarder
    SEE: boarder baby

baby, exceptionally large
    SEE: exceptionally large baby

baby, sick
    SEE: sick baby

BAC
    blood alcohol concentration

backlog
    Claims that have been submitted to the payer but not yet adjudicated.

bad debt
    Charges from patient accounts that are removed from ledgers and "written off" as unpaid after repeated attempts to collect from the patient or insurance carrier.

bad debt ratio
    The proportion of gross revenue that is uncollectable; an indication of effectiveness of billing and collections.

balance billing
    The practice by providers of charging patients the difference between what the payor or insurer reimburses for services and the provider's fee.

bankruptcy
    A legal process that provides an individual or organization protection against creditors while an attempt is made to satisfy debts, either through a financial restructuring or liquidation of assets.
    SEE: Chapter 7
           Chapter 11

bare-bones policy
An affordable health benefit plan with limited coverage, high deductibles, and large copayments.
SYN: no-frills policy

bariatric medicine
The branch of medicine concerned with the treatment of obesity.

baseline
Data about the patient's condition acquired before the initiation of medical care.

base plan
SEE: basic benefit package

base-plus plan
A health benefit design that provides basic coverage and also covers catastrophic injury or illness.

base premium rate
The lowest premium rate for a class of business or a standard package of benefit coverage.

base sanitation
A specified dollar amount allocated to cover health care costs of an insured individual, exclusive of mental health/substance abuse services, pharmacy and administrative charges.

base unit
A service or procedure used to develop a relative value scale for reimbursement.
SEE ALSO: relative value scale

base year
A fiscal year that is used for comparison purposes in the calculation of Medicare costs.

base year costs
The amount of money a hospital paid to care for Medicare patients during a previous time period.

basic benefit package
The portion of a health care benefit plan that provides basic coverage for hospital stays and medical/surgical services.
SYN: base plan
benchmark benefit package
core benefit package
defined benefit package
standard benefit package

basic health services
Health benefits required by federal law of all HMOs.

BB
blood banking

BC
Blue Cross

BCBS
Blue Cross Blue Shield

BCBSA
Blue Cross Blue Shield Association

BCP
biochemistry panel

BE
1. broncho-esophagology
2. barium enema

BEC
behavioral emergency committee

bed capacity
The total number of inpatient beds licensed in a hospital.

bed complement
The number of inpatient beds normally available in a hospital.

bed count day, inpatient
SEE: inpatient bed count day

bed occupancy day
> *SEE:* inpatient service day

bed pan mutual
> An informal term used to denote a physician-owned insurance company.

BEDS
> benefits, evaluations, and data standards

behavior modification
> Strategies intended to change habits that affect health, such as smoking or dieting.

behavior offset
> A decrease in fees paid to physicians during the transition to a fee schedule, such as the resource-based relative value system (RBRVS). Intended to reduce the effect of increased utilization during the transition period.
> *SEE ALSO:* volume adjustment

behavioral emergency committee (BEC)
> An advisory panel based at a hospital that reviews the need for involuntary commitment, restraints or seclusion among patients who may pose a threat to themselves or others.

benchmark
> A standard to which an activity, performance, operation or result is compared.
> *SYN:* reference

benchmark benefit package
> *SEE:* basic benefit package

beneficiary
> A person entitled to receive benefits, such as health coverage. The beneficiary may be the participant, subscriber, or a dependent.
> *SYN:* eligible individual
> *SEE ALSO:* enrollee
> member
> participant
> subscriber

beneficiary, qualified
>   *SEE:* qualified beneficiary

benefit
> The amount of money that may be paid by a health plan for covered health services, or in the case of disability benefits directly to the insured individual.

benefit, alternate
>   *SEE:* alternate benefit

benefit booklet
> Printed material given to subscribers that explains health benefit coverage and provisions in general terms.
>   *SYN:* benefit plan summary
>   *SEE ALSO:* summary plan description

benefit-cost ratio
>   *SEE:* cost-benefit ratio

benefit, daily
>   *SEE:* daily benefit

benefit design
>   *SEE:* benefit package

benefit, lifetime disability
>   *SEE:* lifetime disability benefit

benefit limitation
> Any provision other than an exclusion which restricts health care benefits, regardless of medical necessity. Example: a maximum benefit payable per calendar year for mental health services.

benefit maximum
> The most a health benefit policy will pay for an expense or category of care, expressed in terms of a dollar amount of length of hospitalization.

benefit package
> A set of insurance policy provisions addressing coverage of services, deductibles, and copayments.
>   *SYN:* benefit design

benefit payment schedule
A list that defines the amount of money a benefit plan pays for covered health care services.
SEE ALSO: fee schedule

benefit period
1. The period of time in which benefits are available.
2. The period of time in which deductibles are applied for a health benefit policy. When a new benefit period begins, deductibles must be met again.

benefit plan summary
A general written description of health benefits required by ERISA regulations to be given to employees.
SYN: summary plan description
SEE ALSO: ERISA

benefits, allocated
SEE: allocated benefits

benefits, assignment of
SEE: assignment of benefits

benefits, coordination of
SEE: coordination of benefits

benefits, disability
SEE: disability benefits

benefits, evaluations and data standards (BEDS)

benefits, explanation of
SEE: explanation of benefits

benefits, extension of
SEE: extension of benefits

benefits, indemnity
SEE: indemnity benefits

benefits, loss of income
SEE: disability benefits

benefits, mandated
  SEE: mandated benefits

benefits, portable
  SEE: portable benefits

benefits, qualified
  SEE: qualified benefits

benefits, service
  SEE: service benefits

benefit, unallocated
  SEE: unallocated benefit

benefit year
  A 12-month period used by employers and other groups for the administration of health benefits.

benign
  Referring to a condition that is mild, innocuous, or noncancerous.

b.i.d.
  twice a day

billed charges
  The amount invoiced for medical services under a fee-for-service plan.

billing, direct
  SEE: direct billing

binding arbitration
  Resolution of a dispute, for example a disagreement over a contract, in which both sides agree to abide by a determination made by a disinterested third party.

biofeedback
  Techniques used to gain control over autonomic body functions, such as blood pressure, heart rate, and respiration. Commonly involves the performance of relaxation exercises while a device or machine monitors body functions.

biological
Referring to living organisms and their products.

biological death
Irreversible death of body tissues.
SEE ALSO: clinical death

biopsy
1. The process of obtaining a sample of tissue for diagnostic examination.
2. A sample removed for diagnostic examination.

biorhythm
A cyclic variation in biological function, such as the sleep cycle or circadian rhythms.

biostatistics
The application of the science of statistics to biological or medical data.

birth injury fund
A compensation fund established in many states to compensate patients who suffer permanent injury during birth, as a means of reforming malpractice litigation.

birth on arrival (BOA)
The delivery of a neonate while en route to the hospital.
SYN: en route

birth rate
The number of live births per 1,000 women.

birth weight
The weight of a neonate measured as soon as feasible after delivery, usually expressed in grams.

birth, extramural
SEE: extramural birth

birth, live
SEE: live birth

birthday rule
A provision to determine the primary payer when an individual or family are covered by more than one health benefit plan. According to the birthday rule, the primary payer is the benefit plan of the eligible person whose date of birth falls first in the calendar year, regardless of who is older.
SEE ALSO: coordination of benefits

birthing center
SEE: childbirth center

births, multiple
SEE: multiple births

blacklisting
The practice of avoiding or refusing to insure certain high-risk populations, such as workers in risky industries or occupations.
SEE ALSO: redlining

blue book
A price guide for prescription medication.

blue rules
Policies or regulations that may be modified or violated if necessary.
SEE ALSO: red rules

BM
1. black male
2. bowel movement

BMR
basal metabolic rate

BOA
birth on arrival

board and care facility
A facility that provides lodging, meals, and personal services such as housekeeping for the elderly or those recovering from illness or injury, but not intensive health care services.
SEE ALSO: assisted living facility

board certified
> The designation of a physician who has passed the examination of a recognized medical specialty board.
> > *SYN:* boarded
> > *SEE ALSO:* board eligibility
> > > board eligibility diplomate

boarded
> *SEE:* board certified

board eligible
> The designation of a physician who has completed the education, training, and practice standards required before one is permitted to complete the examination of a medical specialty board.
> > *SEE ALSO:* board certification

boarder
> *SEE:* hospital boarder

boarder baby
> An infant who receives custodial care in a hospital but is not in need of medical care. The parents may be unable or unwilling to assume custody of the infant, who remains in the hospital until a disposition can be made.
> > *SEE ALSO:* hospital border

boarder census
> The number of people receiving meals at a hospital.

board, room and
> *SEE:* room and board

body fluids
> 1. Liquid substances found within or between cells.
> 2. Blood and its constituents, urine, feces, vomitus, saliva, semen and other liquids.

bodywork
> Forms of alternative medicine involving massage, movement, or other types of physical therapies.

booklet, benefit
> *SEE:* benefit booklet

border, hospital
>   *SEE:* hospital border

botanical medicine
>   *SEE:* herbal medicine

BP
blood pressure

BPH
1. benign prostatic hyperplasia
2. benign prostatic hypertrophy

brain death
The absence of cerebral function following cessation of circulation and breathing. Marked by the lack of response to stimulation, the absence of reflexes, the inability to breathe independently, and a flat electroencephalogram for at least 30 minutes.
>   *SYN:* cerebral death
>   *SEE ALSO:* biological death
>   clinical death

break-even point
The level of HMO membership at which revenues and expenses are equal.

bronchoscope
A flexible instrument used to visually inspect the airway.

bronchoscopy
The visual inspection of the airway passages of the lungs.

BRP
bathroom privileges

BS
1. blood sugar
2. Blue Shield

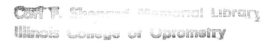

BSN
bachelor of science in nursing

budget
1. A detailed financial plan of income and expenses related to a health care service or program within a specified period of time, usually a year.
2. An amount of money allocated for a project or program.

budget, cash
 SEE: cash budget

budget, global
 SEE: global budget

budget, total
 SEE: global budget

budgeting, capital
 SEE: capital budgeting

BUN
 blood urea nitrogen

bundled
1. The offering of several health benefit plans by one payer.
2. The grouping of codes related to a procedure on a submitted claim.

bundling
 The grouping together of related health care goods and services for the purposes of billing and reimbursement, such as hospital charges and physician fees.
 SYN: global pricing
 SEE ALSO: unbundling

bundling, outpatient
 SEE: outpatient bundling

burn care
 Specialized medical care to patients with severe burns.

burn unit
 A specialized hospital area for the treatment of patients with severe burns.

business insurance

An insurance policy to indemnify losses experienced by a corporate entity, such as a group practice or hospital, rather than an individual.

Bx

biopsy

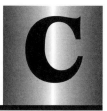

C
celsius, or centigrade

CA
cancer

CABG
coronary artery bypass graft

CAD
1. computer-assisted diagnosis
2. coronary artery disease

cadaver graft
Transplantation of tissue harvested from a deceased donor.

cafeteria plan
SEE: zero-balanced reimbursement account

call
The practice of one physician providing coverage for another during off-hours, such as seeing patients.
SYN: on call

call schedule
The schedule of physician coverage for after-hours care.

CAM
catchment area management

candystriper
SEE: volunteer

cap
1. abbreviation for capsule
2. A maximum limit placed on the expenditure of money for a specific purpose, such as the maximum benefit coverage under a health plan.

cap, out-of-pocket
>*SEE:* out-of-pocket cap

cap, pain and suffering
>*SEE:* pain and suffering cap

capacity
>1. The ability of a health care system to accommodate the demands of routine, after-hours and emergency services.
>2. The number of beds in a hospital.

capital
>Funds for investment in the construction or renovation of facilities, infrastructure and operations.

capital budgeting
>The planning, allocation of funds, and monitoring of investment in major assets, usually fixed assets.

capital expenditure
>An outlay of money to pay for a fixed asset, such as a building or large piece of equipment, that will generate value or benefits over a period of time.

capital expenditure review (CER)

capitation
>Payment of medical services on a flat rate per patient instead of fee-for-service, typically prospectively. Payment is made on a periodic basis, e.g., monthly. Used in health maintenance organizations.
>>*SEE ALSO:* fee-for-service
>>health maintenance organization
>>prospective payment

capitation, risk-adjusted
>*SEE:* risk-adjusted capitation

cardiac arrest
>The sudden cessation of effective cardiac function.
>>*SYN:* full arrest
>>*SEE ALSO:* clinical death

cardiac care unit (CCU)
A hospital unit with specialized facilities, staff and equipment to care for patients who are acutely ill with heart conditions.

cardiac rehabilitation
A program to assist patients recovering from heart attack and other cardiac disorders to improve physical conditioning and cope with the normal physical demands of daily life.

cardiologist
A physician who specializes in the nonsurgical treatment of heart and vascular disorders.

cardiology
The nonsurgical treatment of heart and vascular disease.

cardiopulmonary arrest
SEE: clinical death

cardiovascular
Referring to the heart and blood vessels.

cardiovascular surgeon
A surgeon who specializes in the treatment of heart and vascular conditions.

cardiovascular surgery
The surgical treatment of disorders of the heart and vascular system.

care
1. Treatment and other health services provided for the well-being of one or more patients.
2. The application of knowledge for the benefit of an individual or community.
   SEE ALSO: health care
   service

care, chronic
SEE: chronic care

care, colostomy
SEE: colostomy care

care, continuing
> *SEE:* continuing care

care, custodial
> *SEE:* custodial care

care, domiciliary
> *SEE:* nursing home

care, extended
> *SEE:* extended care

caregiver
> A family member or other person who provides nonmedical care for an ill or disabled individual, such as bathing, feeding and dressing.

care, inpatient
> *SEE:* inpatient care

care, long-term
> *SEE:* long-term care

care manager
> *SEE:* gatekeeper

care, palliative
> *SEE:* palliative care

care, pharmaceutical
> *SEE:* pharmaceutical care

care plan
> *SEE:* nursing care plan

care plan, nursing
> *SEE:* nursing care plan

care, population-based
> *SEE:* population-based care

care, preventive
> *SEE:* preventive care

care, primary
 SEE: primary care

care process models
 SEE: treatment protocol

care, respite
 SEE: respite care

care, secondary
 SEE: specialty care

care, specialty
 SEE: specialty care

care, standard of
 SEE: standard of care

care, subacute
 SEE: subacute care

care, succession of
 SEE: succession of care

care, tertiary
 SEE: tertiary care

care tracks
 SEE: treatment protocol

care, uncompensated
 SEE: uncompensated care

care, unnecessary
 SEE: unnecessary care

care, urgent
 SEE: urgent care

care, well-baby
 SEE: well-baby care

CARF
 Commission on Accreditation of Rehabilitation Facilities

carrier
1. A company that assumes risk by underwriting insurance.
2. A company or agency that underwrites or administers health benefits.
3. An asymptomatic person infected by a contagious disease.
   SYN: insurer
   SEE ALSO: intermediary
               third-party payor

carrier, commercial
SEE: commercial carrier

carrier, indemnity
SEE: indemnity carrier

carve-out
1. A benefit plan addressing a single health care service, e.g., podiatry, pharmaceutical drugs, dental or eye care, or substance abuse and mental health treatment.
2. A disreputable and sometimes illegal scheme of underwriting low-risk healthy employees while higher-risk persons are denied coverage or forced to purchase more expensive policies.
3. A method by which a health plan calculates its secondary liability to Medicare for retirees over the age of 65 by subtracting Medicare's payment from the amount that would have been paid by the health plan had it been designated as primary payer.

case care coordination
SEE: treatment protocol

case management
The ongoing review of patient care by a professional to ensure that services are necessary, appropriate, and cost-effective.

case management, catastrophic
SEE: catastrophic case management

case manager
A professional who reviews patient care to determine the appropriateness and necessity of medical services, and certifies care on an ongoing basis.

case mix
The categorization of patients on the basis of diagnosis.

case-mix index (CMI)
A measure of the relative cost of treatment in an inpatient facility. For example, a case-mix index of .95 means that the treatment of patients in a facility costs 5% below average.

case rate
The payment of a flat fee for all services related to the treatment of a patient based on the diagnosis or presenting problems.

cash budget
An accounting of cash receipts and expenditures used as a short-term financial planning tool.

cash flow
Money paid or received by an organization.

cash indemnity benefits
Money paid by an insurance company to the insured, which may be assigned or transferred to health care providers.

CAT
computed axial tomography
SYN: CAT scan

CAT scan
SEE: computed axial tomography

catastrophic case management
The ongoing review of the appropriateness of services provided to patients with extremely costly medical conditions.
SYN: large case management

catastrophic claim
A request for health benefits to cover a severe illness or injury that is anticipated to involve a long period of treatment and recovery and extraordinary health care costs.

catastrophic coverage
A health benefit policy that provides minimal coverage for health care expenses under a specified level, such as $5,000 a year, but provides coverage for severe and prolonged illness or

injury, ones likely to cause severe financial hardship for the patient.

SYN: catastrophic health insurance

SEE ALSO: basic benefits

major medical

catastrophic health care

Medical services for serious, long-term, or expensive conditions that risk depleting a family's income and resources.

catastrophic health insurance

SEE: catastrophic coverage

catastrophic illness

A severe injury or disease that results in very high expenses, also usually involving a longer duration of health care.

catchment area

A geographic area served by a facility, service, organization or program.

SEE ALSO: health service area

catchment area management (CAM)

categories, ambulatory surgery

SEE: ambulatory surgery categories

categories, major diagnostic

SEE: major diagnostic categories

cause fatality rate

The number of deaths of a specific condition or disease among all reported cases. Usually expressed in terms of deaths per 1,000 or 10,000 cases.

CBC

complete blood count

CBO

Congressional Budget Office

CBP

comprehensive benefit package

cc
  cubic centimeter

CC
  1. cardiac catheterization
  2. chief complaint

CCC
  care, custody and control

CCM
  critical care medicine

CCN
  community care network

CCP
  community care plan

CCRC
  continuing care retirement community

CCU
  1. cardiac care unit
  2. critical care unit

CD
  1. cardiovascular diseases
  2. chemical dependency

CDC
  Centers for Disease Control

CDS
  cardiovascular surgery

CDT
  Current Dental Terminology

CE
  cardiac electrophysiology

cellular therapy
  SEE: live cell therapy

census
The number of patients or residents present in a hospital or other inpatient facility at a given time.

census, average
SEE: average daily census

census, average daily
SEE: average daily census

census, daily
SEE: daily census

census day
SEE: inpatient services day

census, inpatient
SEE: inpatient census

census, boarder
SEE: boarder census

center, birthing
SEE: childbirth center

center, childbirth
SEE: childbirth center

center, outpatient surgery
SEE: outpatient surgery center

centers of excellence
A network of health care facilities and providers selected for their expertise in complicated, sophisticated procedures, such as transplantation.

center, urgent care
SEE: urgent care center

central service
A department in a hospital that sterilizes, prepares and maintains stocks of medical supplies.
SEE ALSO: ancillary services

CEO
chief executive officer

CER
    capital expenditure review

cerebral death
    SEE: brain death

certificate holder
    The individual who represents a family unit covered by a health benefit plan, usually an employee or a member of a group. Generally used to refer to a subscriber of a traditional indemnity benefit plan.
    SYN: insured
          subscriber

certificate of authority (COA)

certificate of coverage (COC)

certificate of insurance (COI)

certificate of need (CON)
    A document issued by the state government officially acknowledging that a proposed health care service, program or facility meets the needs of providing health care to the population.

certification
    1. Approval for admission to a hospital for a given length of stay.
    2. Recognition granted by an independent agency or professional organization that a person has met specified education and training requirements, and passed tests of knowledge and skills.

certification, admission
    SEE: admission certification

certification, board
    SEE: board certification

certification, preadmission
    SEE: preadmission certification

certified nurse midwife (CNM)

CF
conversion factor

CFO
chief financial officer

CHA
community health authority

CHAMPUS
Civilian Health and Medical Program of the Uniformed Services

CHAMPVA
Civilian Health and Medical Program of the Veterans Administration

CHAP
community health accreditation program

Chapter 7
A form of bankruptcy in which a company's assets are liquidated by a court-appointed trustee to compensate the claims of creditors. The company ceases operation.
SEE ALSO: Chapter 11

Chapter 11
A form of bankruptcy in which a company is shielded from creditors while it reorganizes according to a court-approved plan. The company can continue operation.
SEE ALSO: Chapter 7

charge-based reimbursement
A method of health care compensation in which providers are reimbursed at the rate usually charged to all patients. Generally employed with hospitals and other health care facilities.
SYN: charged-based payment system
SEE ALSO: cost-based payment

charges
The dollar amount billed by a health care provider for a service.

charges, allowable
SEE: allowable charges

charges, ancillary
> SEE: ancillary charges

charges, average community
> SEE: average community charges

charges, billed
> SEE: billed charges

charges, covered
> SEE: covered charges

charges, gross
> SEE: gross cost

charges, maximum allowable
> SEE: maximum allowable charges

charges, net
> SEE: net cost

charges, total
> SEE: total charges

charity allowance
A reduction in charges for health services offered to indigent or medically indigent patients.

charity care
Health care services provided without the expectation of receiving payment. Charges are written off because patients have no means to pay.
> SEE: pro bono

CHC
community health center

CHD
coronary heart disease

chelation therapy
Treatment to remove heavy metals, such as mercury and lead, from the body. Chelation therapy is also a form of alternative medicine claimed to reverse atherosclerosis and arteriosclerosis.

chemical dependency (CD)

chemotherapy
The treatment of disease by the administration of chemical agents or other drugs. Often used in association with the treatment of cancer.

cherry-picking
SEE: skimming

CHF
congestive heart failure

chief complaint
The patient's description of symptoms or problems that prompted medical care.

chief executive officer (CEO)
An individual appointed by the governing body of a health care facility or program who is ultimately responsible for its overall operation.

chief financial officer (CFO)
The individual responsible for the overall financial management of a health care facility or entity.

chief of medical staff
SEE: chief of staff

chief of service
A physician who serves as the director or administrative head of a clinical department in a hospital.

chief of staff
A physician who serves as the administrator of the medical staff.
SEE: chief of medical staff

child abuse
The intentional physical or emotional mistreatment of a minor child.

child psychiatrist
A physician who specializes in the evaluation and treatment of children and adolescents with psychiatric disorders.

childbirth center
A hospital-based or freestanding facility specializing in the delivery of newborns, and care of the mothers and infants. Often also provides prenatal and follow-up care for mothers.
SYN: birthing center

childbirth, emergency
SEE: emergency childbirth

CHIN
community health information network

chiropodist
SEE: podiatrist

chiropody
SEE: podiatry

chiropractic
A philosophy of medicine that emphasizes manipulation of the vertebral column.

chiropractor
A practitioner of chiropractic.

CHMIS
community health management information system

CHN
1. child neurology
2. community health network

cholangiogram
An x-ray of the bile duct in which structures are visualized with a dye.

cholecystogram
An x-ray of the gallbladder.

CHP
1. child and adolescent psychiatry
2. comprehensive health planning

chronic
Describing a disease or condition with gradual onset, slow progress and long duration.

chronic care
Health services for individuals with persistent, ongoing conditions. Chronic care not only addresses the underlying condition, but also aims to promote health, encourage self-care and limit disability.

churning
1. A reimbursement system based on the productivity of providers.
2. The practice of seeing a patient more than is medically necessary in order to increase reimbursement from a health care plan.

CIN
cervical intraepithelial neoplasia

circulating nurse
A nurse whose responsibilities as a member of an operating room team are to handle instruments, equipment, and supplies, but usually is not directly involved in surgery.

circulation technologist
SEE: cardiovascular perfusionist

CIS
carcinoma in situ

claim
1. The documentation of services provided under a health benefit plan, which is filed by the provider for payment or reimbursement from the payer.
2. A request for workers' compensation benefits.

claimant
A health plan or workers' compensation beneficiary who files a request for benefits.

claim, closed
> *SEE:* closed claim

claim form
A document used to file for health care benefits.

claim lag
1. The duration between the date a claim is incurred and its payment.
2. The duration between the date a claim is incurred and its submission to the payer.

claims, expected
> *SEE:* expected claims

claims, incurred
> *SEE:* incurred claims

claims manager
An individual employed by the payer to supervise the processing of health care claims.

claims payment fraud
The intentional falsification of information related to treatment or charges that results in a lower payment of health benefits to providers or the insured.

claims reporting fraud
The intentional misrepresentation or falsification of information related to treatment or charges that results in a higher payment of benefits to providers or the insured.

claims review
1. The evaluation of a beneficiaries' health care service claim prior to reimbursement to determine whether care is appropriate and not excessively costly.
2. The evaluation of appropriateness and medical need after a request for health care service has been denied.

classical fee-for-service
The payment of health care services out-of-pocket by the patient or consumer.
> *SEE ALSO:* traditional fee-for-service

clause, exclusivity
SEE: exclusivity clause

clause, hold harmless
SEE: hold harmless clause

clause, no-shop
SEE: no-shop clause

clause, recurring
SEE: recurring clause

clerk, clinic
SEE: clinic clerk

clerk, unit
SEE: unit clerk

clerk, ward
SEE: unit clerk

CLIA
Clinical Laboratory Improvement Act of 1988
SYN: CLIA-88

CLIA-88
SEE: CLIA

CLIAC
Clinical Laboratory Improvement Advisory Committee

clinic
1. An outpatient facility.
2. A medical service, such as pediatrics, organized around specialized medical areas, such as pediatrics.

clinic clerk
A person who performs clerical functions in an outpatient facility or group practice office.

clinic manager
The administrator or chief executive officer of an outpatient facility.

clinic, satellite
SEE: satellite clinic

clinic without walls (CWW)
A corporate organization in which physicians or other providers maintain their own practice offices but have centralized management facilities for billing, staffing, marketing, and other business services.

clinical
Related to the care of human patients.

clinical algorithm
SEE: treatment protocol

clinical death
The cessation of respiration and cardiac function. May be reversed by resuscitation.
SYN: cardiac arrest
SEE: biological death
brain death
cardiopulmonary arrest
full arrest

clinical diagnosis
The determination of the nature of a disease on the basis of its signs and symptoms, combined with a physical examination and the results of laboratory and radiologic diagnostic tests.

clinical ecology
SEE: environmental medicine

clinical guidelines
SEE: treatment protocol

clinical integration
1. The creation of relationships among different types of medical providers (i.e., physicians, hospitals, and health plans) to enhance the coordination of patient care.
2. The creation of a single medical record accessible to all health service providers involved in the care of a patient.

clinical investigator
An individual who conducts research involving patients, often funded by grants from the federal government, medical or pharmaceutical companies.

clinical outcome
The status of a patient's health after medical treatment.

clinical pathway
A set of guidelines incorporating algorithms and the process of decision tree analysis to assist in the proper diagnosis and treatment of illnesses, injuries, or conditions.
SYN: critical pathway
SEE: treatment protocol

clinical privileges
Authority granted to a physician or other health professional to admit patients to a medical facility.

clinical privileging
The review and evaluation of a provider's credentials for the purposes of granting the right to operate within a health care facility or organization.
SYN: credentialing

clinical protocols
SEE: treatment protocol

clinical research
Scientific study or experimentation involving human patients.

clinical resume
SEE: discharge summary

clinical roadmap
The allocation of health care resources to provide the optimal level of service to a group of patients, with an emphasis on prevention, early diagnosis, and management of chronic illness.

clinical service
1. A unit or department of medical providers within a health care organization or facility, such as pediatrics.
2. A unit of inpatient beds in a medical facility.

3. A group of patients with related conditions or treatments.

4. The delivery of health care to patients.

clinical subspecialty
> *SEE:* subspecialty

clinical trial
> An experimental process involving human patients to evaluate the efficacy or safety of a new drug or procedure.

clinical trial, phase I
> *SEE:* phase I clinical trial

clinical trial, phase II
> *SEE:* phase II clinical trial

clinical trial, phase III
> *SEE:* phase III clinical trial

clinician
> A general term denoting a medical professional who cares for patients, as opposed to one who primarily works in a laboratory, for example.

closed claim
> A claim for which all benefits have been paid.

closed panel
> The delivery of health care services by a limited network or group of providers. Providers may be employees of an HMO or independent providers under contract to serve the HMO exclusively. Eligible patients receive benefits only when care is received from a provider who belongs to the network.
> *SYN:* group model HMO
> *SEE ALSO:* open panel
> staff model HMO

closed staff
> A network of providers that does not accept new patients.

closed surgery
> An operative procedure performed with needles or endoscopic instruments, without large incisions in the skin to expose internal structures.
> *SEE ALSO:* minimally invasive surgery

closing date
The date identified in a master agreement on which a transaction is consummated.

CLP
clinical pathology

cm
centimeter

CM
1. case management
2. case manager

CME
continuing medical education

CMHC
community mental health center

CMI
case mix index

CMP
1. chemical pathology
2. comprehensive medical plan

CMSA
Case Management Society of America

CNM
certified nurse midwife

CNS
central nervous system

c/o
complains of

COA
certificate of authority

COB
coordination of benefits

COBRA
Consolidated Omnibus Budget Reconciliation Act of 1985; requires employers offering group health plans to allow terminated employees and their dependents to continue coverage for a period of time on a self-pay basis.

COC
certificate of coverage

code blue
A term often used in hospital paging systems to signal an emergency, such as cardiac arrest, to members of a resuscitation team.

code creep
Invoicing for procedures or physician services that were not performed, or are charges at a level higher than the procedure actually performed.
SEE ALSO: overbilling
overcoding

code, CPT
SEE: current procedural terminology

coding
The classification of principal and related diagnoses into a numerical designation.

cohort study
A clinical investigation in which a group is chosen for a common characteristic (e.g., age or diagnosis) during a period of time.

COI
certificate of insurance

coinsurance, co-insurance
The portion of the cost of health benefits paid by the individual, usually a percentage of the total cost or amount approved by the payer.
SEE ALSO: copayment

cold therapy
> *SEE:* cryotherapy

collaboration
> The commitment of two or more individuals or entities to work cooperatively toward an agreed-upon goal.

collaborative care tracks
> *SEE:* treatment protocol

collaborative case management plans
> *SEE:* treatment protocol

collaborative paths
> *SEE:* treatment protocol

colon and rectal surgery
> A medical/surgical specialty involving the diagnosis and treatment of conditions affecting the lower intestinal tract, including colon, rectum, and adjacent areas.
> *SYN:* proctology

colon therapy
> A form of alternative medicine that claims to cleanse or detoxify the body by enemas.

colonoscope
> An instrument used to visually inspect the interior of the colon.
> *SEE:* endoscope

colonoscopy
> The visual examination of the interior of the colon with a colonoscope.

color healing
> *SEE:* color therapy

color therapy
> A form of alternative medicine that claims a therapeutic effect by color and light.
> *SYN:* color healing

colorectal
> Referring to the colon and rectum.

colorectal surgery
> *SEE:* colon and rectal surgery

colostomy
> The creation by surgery of an opening between the colon and the abdominal wall, which diverts waste products to the body surface.

colostomy care
> Specialized nursing and medical services for patients with a colostomy.

come-and-go surgery
> *SEE:* ambulatory surgery

commercial carrier
> A health insurance company operated on a for-profit basis.

committee, joint study
> *SEE:* joint study committee

communicable disease
> An illness capable of transmission from person to person or from animal to human, i.e., an infectious disease.
> *SYN:* contagious disease

community-based services
> Health care, mental health, social work and other services that are located in local clinics or outpatient facilities. Although affiliated with a medical center, community-based services are not typically housed in a hospital.

community health
> Activities, services, and programs intended to improve the health conditions of a specific community.
> *SYN:* public health

community health accreditation program (CHAP)

community health authority (CHA)

community health care
Health services designed to improve the well-being of community residents.
SEE ALSO: public health

community health center (CHC)

community health information network (CHIN)
An integrated network of computers and electronic systems linking multiple providers, payers, employers, and other health care entities within a geographic region. Permits the exchange of clinical, administrative and financial information among members of the network.
SYN: community health management information system

community health management information system (CHMIS)

community health network (CHN)

community hospital
A medical facility, often operated on a non-profit basis, dedicated to serving the health care needs of a neighborhood or community. Typically provides less intensive services than a tertiary care facility, with more of an emphasis on primary care and preventive medicine.

community mental health center (CMHC)
A facility and staff that provides mental health services on an outpatient basis to individuals who live or work in defined catchment areas. In general, the aim of a community mental health center is to avoid hospitalization through counseling, crisis intervention, medication management, and vocational rehabilitation.

community rating
Pricing insurance based on the average cost of providing benefits for all persons within a defined geographic area, without adjusting for an individual's demographic characteristics, medical history or likelihood of using health care services.
SEE ALSO: adjusted community rating
experience rating
modified community rating

community rating, modified
  SEE: modified community rating

community, life-care
  SEE: life-care community

comorbid condition
  SEE: comorbidity

comorbidity
  1. The simultaneous existence of two or more unrelated diseases.
  2. The presence of a comorbid condition at the time of admission to a hospital can be expected to increase health care costs and the length of hospital stay.
  SYN: comorbid condition
     substantial comorbidity

company, insurance
  SEE: insurance company

company, limited liability
  SEE: limited liability company

comparability provision
  A regulation specifying that reasonable charges for health services under Medicare cannot be greater than comparable services charged to non-Medicare patients covered by private insurance.

compensation fund
  A reserve created by contributions from providers, insurers, and hospitals to compensate patients injured in the course of medical care.
  SEE ALSO: alternative dispute resolution

competency, cultural
  SEE: cultural competency

competition, managed
  SEE: managed competition

compliance
   The degree to which a patient follows a treatment regimen
   prescribed by a physician or other health care provider.
   SYN: patient compliance
   SEE ALSO: non-compliance

complication
   1. A process or event occurring during the course of an illness
      that worsens a patient's condition.
   2. A condition arising during hospitalization that increases the
      patient's stay in 75% of the cases.

composite rate
   A premium rate applied to all persons enrolled in a group benefit plan, regardless of the number of dependents. A feature
   sometimes seen in large employer groups and unions.

comprehensive health planning (CHP)

comprehensive major medical insurance
   A health benefit plan that provides coverage offered in a basic
   plan and a major medical health insurance policy. Typically
   features a low deductible, coinsurance and high maximum
   benefits.

computed axial tomography (CAT)

CON
   certificate of need

concurrent review
   The assessment of health care processes and outcomes during a
   patient's course of treatment.
   SEE ALSO: prospective review
                retrospective review

condition, critical
   SEE: critical condition

condition, pre-existing
   SEE: pre-existing condition

conference, clinical
   SEE: clinical conference

confidentiality
The right of patients to have information about their health, such as the medical record, disclosed without consent.

confidentiality agreement
A contract between parties of a proposed transaction to agree that information shared among them will remain confidential.

consent, implied
SEE: implied consent

consent, imposed
SEE: imposed consent

consolidation
1. A transaction in which the assets and operations of two organizations are combined into a single new corporation.
2. The regrouping of programs or services.
SEE ALSO: merger

consolidation, financial
SEE: financial consolidation

consortium
A formal organization of independent groups or institutions working together in collaborative projects or joint ventures.

consult
A specialist who performs an evaluation at the request of a primary care physician.

consultant, outside
SEE: outside consultant

consultation
An evaluation and recommendation by a specialist at the request of a primary care physician.
SYN: consult

contagion
The transmission of disease by contact with a sick person.

contagious disease
SEE: communicable disease

contingency reserve, physician
>   *SEE:* physician contingency reserve

continued stay review (CSR)
>   The evaluation of a patient's medical record to determine the medical necessity of remaining in the hospital.

continuing care
>   The provision of a comprehensive range of health services over a period of time, including skilled nursing care, intermediate care and hospice care, in a variety of settings.

continuing-care retirement community (CCRC)
>   A residential arrangement that offers a range of housing options for elderly persons, from apartments for independent residents, to assisted-living facilities and extended-care facilities. Provides a continuum of care for the varying needs of the aging person.

continuing medical education (CME)

contract
>   1. A legal agreement between two or more individuals or entities.
>   2. An agreement between an insurer or HMO and a subscriber group which specifies premium rates, benefits, limitations, and other conditions.

contract fee schedule plan
>   A health benefit plan in which providers agree to accept a schedule of specific fees as the total charges for care, procedures or services rendered.

contract, group
>   *SEE:* group contract

contract mix
>   The categorization of enrollees in terms of dependents, i.e., individual coverage, husband and wife, or family. Used to determine average contract size.

contract practice
>   An individual provider or a group of providers who contract directly with self-insured employers or third-party administrators to supply health care services.
>   *SEE ALSO:* direct contracting

contract provider
A physician, hospital, facility, agency or individual who has a contractual agreement with a payer to provide health care goods and services.

contract term
The period of time for which a contract is written, usually 12 months.

contract year
Twelve consecutive months following the anniversary date of a contract. May or may not coincide with the calendar year.

contracted management organization
An organization that supplies billing, collection or other management support services for independent provider practices.

contracting, direct
  SEE: direct contracting

contractual allowances
Adjustments resulting from agreements between providers and third party payers, such as Medicare and Medicaid.
  SYN: purchase discount

contribution, equal-dollar
  SEE: equal-dollar contribution

contribution, equal-percentage
  SEE: equal-percentage contribution

contributory plan
A health benefit plan in which the covered individual shares in the cost of premiums, usually through a periodic payroll deduction.
  SEE ALSO: non-contributory plan

contributory premium
The portion of a health benefit plan premium that is paid by the insured or member.

convalescent care
 SEE: extended care

convalescent care facility
 SEE: extended care facility

conversion factor (CF)
 Under the resource-based relative value system (RBRVS) of compensation a dollar amount multiplied by the relative value schedule (RVS) of a procedure to determine the maximum allowable amount.
 SEE ALSO: maximum allowable
    relative value schedule
    resource-based relative value system

conversion privilege
 The right of a person covered by a group health plan to continue coverage as an individual after the termination of employment.

COO
 chief operating officer

cookbook medicine
 An informal term for health care that follows explicit treatment guidelines or protocols.
 SEE ALSO: treatment protocol

coordinated care
 SEE: treatment protocol

coordination of benefits (COB)
 A process employed when a patient is covered by more than one health benefit plan to determine which plan is primary and to ensure that payments are not in excess of the charges for services rendered.
 SEE ALSO: birthday rule

copay, co-pay
 SEE: copayment

copayment, co-payment
A predetermined fee paid by the patient directly to the provider for a product or service, such as an office visit or prescription medication. Intended to limit utilization of health services,
SYN: copay
surcharge

COPCP
community-oriented primary care program

COPD
chronic obstructive pulmonary disease

core benefit package
SEE: basic benefit package

core coverage
Basic medical benefits, excluding services such as vision and dental care.
SEE ALSO: non-core coverage

CORF
comprehensive outpatient rehabilitation facility

corporate alliance
SEE: alliance

corporation, dental service
SEE: dental service corporation

corporation, service
SEE: service corporation

corrective action
Steps to remedy an identified problem.

cosmetic surgery
An elective surgical procedure primarily to enhance a patient's appearance.
SEE ALSO: elective surgery
medically necessary

cost-based payment

A system of compensating providers based on the actual costs of providing care, according to guidelines established by third-party payers. Employed most often by hospitals and other health care facilities.

SYN: retrospective reimbursement

SEE ALSO: charge-based reimbursement

cost-benefit ratio

An way of analyzing expenditures, determined by dividing the value of cash revenue by the value of the investment required of the project. a ratio of less than one is usually considered unacceptable.

SYN: benefit-cost ratio

cost center

An accounting method to segregate and record all costs associated with a department, program service or activity.

cost containment

Strategies to reduce or eliminate unnecessary and costly medical services.

SEE ALSO: managed care

cost-efficiency

1. The production of goods or services at the least possible cost.
2. The treatment of a medical condition with the least expensive level of care that achieves the desired health outcome of the patient.

SEE ALSO: efficiency

cost, fixed

SEE: fixed cost

cost of living rider

A provision sometimes included in a disability benefit policy that increases monthly payments during the claim to account for inflation.

cost outlier
A patient whose medical care is significantly more expensive than other patients with a similar condition.

cost reimbursement
A method of compensating providers based on the actual costs incurred in the delivery of health goods and services.

cost sharing
Money paid by patients for health care services covered by a health benefit plan, including contributory premiums, deductibles, co-payments and coinsurance. Provides financial disincentive against the utilization of services.
Syn: out-of-pockets
See also: contributory plan
out-of-pocket expenses

cost-shifting
The practice among providers of increasing health care charges billed to patients with generous health benefit plans to make up revenue lost on managed care contracts.

costs
The dollar amount incurred by providing a health care service.

costs, administrative
See: administrative costs

costs, base year
See: base year costs

costs, out-of-pocket
See: out-of-pocket costs

costs, variable
See: variable costs

cost, variable
See: variable cost

courtesy, professional
See: professional courtesy

coverage
The type and amount of benefits provided by a health plan.

coverage, catastrophic
SEE: catastrophic coverage

coverage, core
SEE: core coverage

coverage, first-dollar
SEE: first-dollar coverage

coverage, non-core
SEE: non-core coverage

covered benefits
Medically necessary health care services available to an eligible person under a benefit program.
SYN: covered services

covered charges
Charges for health care services and goods that qualify as covered benefits and are paid in part or in whole by a health benefit plan. May be affected by deductibles, copayments, and annual or lifetime maximums.

covered lives
The number of persons, including dependents, who are eligible for benefits in a health plan.

covered person
An individual eligible for benefits under a health benefit plan.
SYN: eligible

covered services
Health care services for which benefits are provided under the terms of a health benefit contract.
SEE ALSO: covered benefits

CP
1. cerebral palsy
2. chest pain

CPD
cephalopelvic disproportion

CPI
consumer price index

CPI-MCS
consumer price index — medical care services

CPO
contract provider organization

CPR
1. cardiopulmonary resuscitation
2. customary, prevailing and reasonable fees

CPT
current procedural terminology

CPT code
A numerical code assigned to procedures performed by health care providers for the purposes of billing, according to the Current Procedural Terminology (CPT) published by the American Medical Association.
SEE ALSO: current procedural terminology

CPU
central processing unit

CQI
continuous quality improvement

CQMS
cost quality management system

crash cart
A wheeled cabinet or cart containing drugs and equipment used for resuscitation.

CRC
community rating by class

credentialing
A systematic process used by HMOs and other managed care organizations to evaluate the competence and practice patterns of providers. Typically includes such factors as experience, board certification status, measures of clinical practice and other qualifications.
SEE ALSO: board certification
practice pattern analysis
profiling

creditor
A person or corporate entity to whom a debt is owed.

criteria
Endpoints or elements by which the quality and appropriateness of health care can be measured.

criteria, pre-established
SEE: pre-established criteria

criteria, validation
SEE: validation criteria

criterion, validation
SEE: validation criterion

critical pathway
SEE: clinical pathway

CRNA
certified registered nurse anesthetist

CRS
colon and rectal surgery

CRT
cathode ray tube

cryotherapy
Treatment involving the application of cold or freezing temperatures to the body.
SYN: cold therapy

crystal therapy
An alternative medicine that attributes healing properties to gemstones, minerals and crystals.

CS
central services

C&S
culture and sensitivity

CSD
cumulative stress disorder

CSF
cerebrospinal fluid

CSI
computed severity index

CSM
consolidated standards manual

CSR
continued stay review

CST
certified surgical technician

CT
computed tomography

CTD
cumulative trauma disorder

cu mm
cubic millimeter

cultural competency
The recognition and appreciation for differences among ethnic groups and the relationship with the etiology and cultural context of disease.

Current Dental Terminology (CDT)
A list of terms and identifying codes for dental procedures created by the American Dental Association for uniform reporting of dental services and procedures to health benefit plans.

current procedural terminology (CPT)
A standardized system of reporting health services using numeric codes according to a list developed and updated by the American Medical Association.

custodial care
Services that primarily meet personal needs, such as bathing, dressing, eating and taking medications. Typically provided by individuals without medical training.
SEE ALSO: activities of daily living

customary fee
A payable fee level for a specific procedure determined by a health benefit plan administrator based on actual charges for the procedure submitted by a larger group of providers.
SEE ALSO: reasonable fee
usual, customary and reasonable plan
usual fee

CVA
cerebrovascular accident

CVT
cardiovascular technician

CWW
clinic without walls

CXR
chest x-ray

cycle billing
The practice of maintaining cash flow by billing third-party payers a portion of patient statements at specific intervals, usually weekly.

CyP
cytopathology

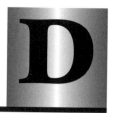

d
> day

D
> 1. day (d)
> 2. dermatology

daily benefit
> The maximum amount payable by a health benefit plan for room and board charges at a hospital.

daily census
> The number of patients present in a health care facility, including patients who were admitted and discharged since the last time the census was completed.
> *SYN:* daily inpatient census

daily census, weighted
> *SEE:* weighted daily census

daily inpatient census
> *SEE:* daily census

daily rate
> *SEE:* per diem

daily recap sheet
> The daily census, plus outpatients, boarders, newborns, and deaths.
> *SEE ALSO:* daily census

daily service charge
> The amount charged for one day of stay in a health care facility.

data, encounter
> *SEE:* encounter data

data retrieval
The gathering of patient care information from medical records.

data set
A collection of uniformly defined elements of information about an aspect of health care.

data sources
Medical records and documents used for the auditing of patient care.

date, admission
   SEE: admission date

date, discharge
   SEE: discharge date

date, eligibility
   SEE: eligibility date

date, expiration
   SEE: expiration date

dates, admission and discharge
   SEE: admission and discharge dates

DATTA
Diagnostic and Therapeutic Technology Assessment Program

DAW
dispense as written

day care, adult
   SEE: adult day care

day, inpatient bed count
   SEE: inpatient bed count day

day, inpatient services
   SEE: inpatient services day

day outlier
   SEE: stay outlier

day, resident
   SEE: resident day

days, discharge
> *SEE:* length of stay

days of revenue in receivables (DRR)
> The average number of days after services are rendered until fees are collected on patient accounts.
> *SYN:* days outstanding

days of stay
> *SEE:* length of stay

days outstanding
> *SEE:* days of revenue in receivables

day surgery
> *SEE:* outpatient surgery

DC
> 1. discharge
> 2. discontinue
> 3. dual choice

D.C.
> Doctor of chiropractic medicine

D&C
> dilation and curettage

DCG
> diagnostic cost group

DCI
> duplicate coverage inquiry

DCP
> dental capitation plan

D.D.S.
> Doctor of dental surgery

DEA
> Drug Enforcement Administration

death
The permanent cessation of all life functions.
SYN: adverse patient outcome
SEE ALSO: biological death
brain death
clinical death

death benefit
An amount of money payable to a designated beneficiary after the death of a person covered by a life insurance policy.

death benefit, accelerated
SEE: accelerated death benefit

death benefit, accidental
SEE: accidental death benefit

death, biological
SEE: biological death

death, clinical
SEE: clinical death

death, wrongful
SEE: wrongful death

debridement
The removal of dead tissue from a wound or burn to prevent infection and promote healing.

declination
The rejection of an applicant for insurance coverage, usually due to reasons of health or other risks.

decontamination
The neutralization or removal of hazardous substances from the environment.
SEE ALSO: disinfection
sterilization

decredentialing
SEE: deselection

deductible
The amount of money a person must pay in plan-approved health care expenses before insurance coverage commences. A cost-sharing arrangement common in traditional indemnity health benefit plans. Members of an HMO usually do not pay deductibles.
SEE ALSO: cost-sharing
out-of-pocket

defined benefit package
SEE: basic benefit package

degeneration
The gradual deterioration of the normal function and structure of cells and tissue.

degenerative disease
An illness in which there is a gradual deterioration of the structure or function of tissue.

deinstitutionalization
The discharge of large number of patients with chronic mental illness who had been previously maintained in long-term facilities. Deinstitutionalization became widespread in the U.S. during the 1970s and 1980s. Although it was believed patients would be maintained at community mental health centers, many dropped out of the system and became homeless.

delivery, normal
SEE: normal delivery

delivery, precipitate
SEE: emergency childbirth

demand
The amount of services sought from a health care system by a population of patients.

dental service corporation
A non-profit organization that administers dental benefit plans, such as the Blue Cross/Blue Shield plans.

dependent
A person other than the insured who is eligible for coverage under a health benefit plan, such as a spouse or a child.

dermatologist
A physician who specializes in the diagnosis and treatment of conditions affecting the skin.

dermatology
The treatment of diseases of the skin.

description, summary plan
SEE: benefit plan summary

deselection
The elimination or dismissal of a provider from a managed care network.
SYN: decredentialing

detox
SEE: detoxification

detoxification
Recovery from the acute effects of poison, drugs, or alcohol.
SYN: detox

developmental delay
SEE: developmental disability

developmental disability
The failure or delay of progression through the normal milestones or due to mental, emotional or physical impairment.
SYN: developmental delay

DHHS
Department of Health and Human Services

diagnosis
The determination of the nature of a patient's illness, injury, or condition.

diagnosis, admission
SEE: admission diagnosis

diagnosis by exclusion
The determination of the nature of an illness by eliminating possible causes that are not consistent with the patient's signs and symptoms.

diagnosis, clinical
SEE: clinical diagnosis

diagnosis, differential
SEE: differential diagnosis

diagnosis, discharge
SEE: discharge diagnosis

diagnosis, dual
SEE: dual diagnosis

diagnosis, laboratory
SEE: laboratory diagnosis

diagnosis, major
SEE: major diagnosis

diagnosis, physical
SEE: physical diagnosis

diagnosis, prenatal
SEE: prenatal diagnosis

diagnosis, principal
SEE: principal diagnosis

diagnosis, provisional
SEE: admission diagnosis

diagnosis-related groups (DRG)
A method of categorizing patients based on a medical grouping by diagnostic categories, for the purposes of reimbursement by payers. Adopted by the Health Care Financing Administration for Medicare patients, and subsequently embraced by insurers, managed care companies and other payers.
SEE ALSO: ambulatory surgery categories
major diagnostic categories

diagnosis, tentative
> *SEE:* admission diagnosis

diagnostic
> Referring to a process, procedure or test intended to provide information about the nature of the patient's condition.

diagnostic services
> Tests, examinations, and procedures performed to determine the nature of the patient's condition.

dialysis
> A procedure employed to filter and remove waste products from the blood when a person suffers from kidney failure.

DIC
> disseminated intravascular coagulation

diener
> A technician who assists the pathologist during an autopsy.
> *SYN:* morgue technician

dietitian, registered
> *SEE:* registered dietitian

differential
> The difference in out-of-pocket expenses an eligible person may pay in choosing between traditional indemnity coverage and a managed care plan.

differential cost
> *SEE:* marginal cost

differential diagnosis
> A short list of possible conditions that may be causing the patient's signs and symptoms, which are then ruled out or confirmed by further evaluation and testing in descending order of seriousness or likelihood.

diligence, due
> *SEE:* due diligence

diplomate
A term sometimes used to describe a physician who is board certified in a medical speciality or subspecialty.
SYN: board certification
board certified
boarded specialty
SEE ALSO: subspecialty

direct billing
The practice of billing patients for the cost of health care services or goods, rather than billing a third-party payer.

direct contracting
Arrangements for health services made between employers and providers without the use of an insurer or health maintenance organization. Usually covered by ERISA regulations.
SEE ALSO: ERISA

directed imagery
SEE: imagery

direct pay
The continuation of health benefit coverage on a private basis after a member's group coverage is terminated.

direct payment subscriber
An individual enrolled in a health maintenance organization who pays a premium directly to the HMO rather than through a group. Typically, the cost to the individual are greater and benefits are less extensive then under a group plan.

direct reimbursement
A self-funded health benefit plan that pays to eligible individuals a percentage of the actual cost of care that is received. Typically, beneficiaries are free to seek care from a provider of their choice.

disability
An impairment or loss of function.
SEE ALSO: permanent disability
temporary disability

disability benefit, lifetime
> *SEE:* lifetime disability benefit

disability benefits
> Payments compensating for lost income to an insured individual who is unable to work due to a covered injury or illness.
> *SYN:* disability compensation

disability compensation
> *SEE:* disability benefits

disability, developmental
> *SEE:* developmental disability

disability, learning
> *SEE:* learning disability

disability, long-term
> *SEE:* long-term disability

disability, partial
> *SEE:* partial disability

disability, permanent
> *SEE:* permanent disability

disability, short-term
> *SEE:* short-term disability

disability, total
> *SEE:* total disability

discharge
> The release of a patient from hospitalization.

discharge date
> The calendar date on which a patient is formally released from a health care facility.

discharge days
> *SEE:* length of stay

discharge diagnosis
A diagnosis provided by the attending physician upon the patient's discharge from the hospital. Because the discharge diagnosis is based on observation, laboratory testing and other diagnostic information obtained during hospitalization, it is usually more accurate than the admission diagnosis.

discharge plan
A written plan that identifies the health care needs of a patient and makes provisions for appropriate services following release from hospitalization.

discharges
The number of patients released from a hospital within a given time period.

discharge status
Disposition of the patient upon formal release from a health care facility, i.e., home, extended care facility, etc.

discharge summary
A concise description of the patient's hospitalization entered into the medical record, including the reasons for admission, findings of laboratory testing and other diagnostic procedures, the discharge diagnosis, and instructions for the patient.
SYN: clinical resume

disclosure, fee
SEE: fee disclosure

discounted fee-for-service
The reimbursement of physician services on a fee-for-service basis, but at a rate below usual and customary fees. Used in preferred provider organizations (PPOs) and health maintenance organizations (HMOs).
SEE ALSO: preferred provider organization

disease
A sickness or disorder of normal body function, characterized by a recognized cause and identifiable signs and symptoms
SEE ALSO: syndrome

disease, acute
SEE: acute illness

disease, communicable
SEE: communicable disease

disease, degenerative
SEE: degenerative disease

disease, iatrogenic
SEE: iatrogenic disease

disease management
A coordinated, disease-specific approach to patient care intended to achieve the optimal cost-effective outcome. Involves the full continuum of care, from the identification of a condition to prevention and health maintenance through treatment, follow-up and outcomes measurement.
SYN: disease state management

disease, medically induced
SEE: iatrogenic disease

disease, nosocomial
SEE: nosocomial disease

disease staging
An evaluation of the severity of a disease such as cancer by determining the phases in the course of the disease process.

disease state management
SEE: disease management

disenrollment
Termination of health benefit coverage.
SYN: fall-out

disinfection
The destruction or inhibition of disease-causing microorganisms.
SEE ALSO: decontamination
        sterilization

dispense as written (DAW)
A designation made by a physician in a prescription that directs the pharmacist to fill the order with brand-name medications rather than a generic substitution.

diuretic
SEE: water pill

divestiture
The involuntary sale or exchange subsidiary, such as to comply with federal antitrust laws.
SEE ALSO: spin-off

DJD
degenerative joint disease

DLI
diagnostic laboratory immunology

DMA
Director of medical affairs

DME
1. director of medical education
2. durable medical equipment

DMO
dental maintenance organization

DMS
diagnostic medical sonographer

DMSO
dimethyl sulfoxide

DMSO therapy
The use of dimethyl sulfoxide (DMSO) in the treatment of cancer or other diseases.

DNAR
do not attempt resuscitation

DNR
do-not-resuscitate

DO
Doctor of Osteopathy

doctor
SEE: physician

domiciliary care
SEE: nursing home

domiciliary care facility
A residential facility that provides lodging, meals and personal services for the elderly and those with long-term illness, but not health care services.

do-not-resuscitate order (DNR)
Explicit instructions to health care providers that a terminally ill patient is not to be resuscitated in the event of cardiopulmonary arrest.
SEE ALSO: advance directive
living will

DOS
date of service

dose
The quantity of a medication given at once or in fractions over a period of time.
SEE ALSO: dosage
regimen

DOT
Department of Transportation

double indemnity
SEE: accidental death benefit

downcoding
The changing of health benefit billing codes by third-party payers to reflect a procedure that is less complex and/or compensated at a lower rate than what was reported.

DP
dermatopathology

DPA
durable power of attorney

DPM
Doctor of podiatric medicine

DPR
drug price review

dr
dram

DR
diagnostic radiology

drama therapy
The use of theater or drama to achieve therapeutic goals.

DRE
digital rectal exam

dread disease insurance
An insurance policy that provides coverage for medical expenses associated with specified diseases or conditions, such as cancer.

DRG
diagnosis-related group

DRGs, low volume
SEE: low volume DRGs

DRR
days of revenue in receivables

drug therapy, maintenance
SEE: maintenance drug therapy

DSM
Diagnostic and Statistical Manual of Mental Disorders

DSRF
debt service reserve fund

DT
1. dietetic services
2. dietetic technician

DTR
deep tendon reflex

dual choice
SEE: dual option

dual diagnosis
Concomitant mental illness and substance abuse.

dual option
A health benefit design that allows eligible persons more than one choice of financing and delivery systems, such as a health maintenance organization and traditional indemnity coverage.
SYN: dual choice
multiple choice

due diligence
A legal process of investigating the operations and financial condition of a proposed partner, usually prior to a merger or acquisition, to determine and verify the risks of the transaction and the suitability of the organization.

DUM
drug utilization management

dumping
SEE: patient dumping

dumping, patient
SEE: patient dumping

DUR
drug utilization review

durable medical equipment (DME)
Devices and other equipment related to the patient's health care needs in the home, usually intended for long-term repeated use. Includes hospital beds, wheelchairs and other mobility devices, oxygen therapy equipment, and IV therapy equipment.

durable power of attorney (DPA)
A legal document prepared by one person authorizing another to make decisions in the event he or she is incapacitated. May not apply to health care decisions.
SEE ALSO: health care proxy

duration of hospitalization, average
SEE: average duration of hospitalization

duration of inpatient hospitalization
SEE: length of stay

DVT
deep vein thrombosis

DX
diagnosis

DXL
diagnostic x-rays and laboratory

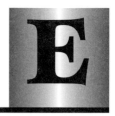

EAP
employee assistance program

EAPA
Employee Assistance Professionals Association

Early and Periodic Screening, Diagnosis and Treatment (EPSDT)
A preventive health program to detect and treat physical and mental problems among patients under the age of 21.

EBIS
employee benefit information system

EBR
1. employee benefit representative
2. employee benefit review

EBRI
Employee Benefits Research Institute

ECF
extended care facility

ECG
electrocardiogram

ECHO
echocardiogram

ECMO
extracorporeal membrane oxygenation

economic integration
A formal relationship among two or more types of health care providers who share joint financial interest in providing medical care and services under contractual arrangements.

ECU
   emergency care unit

ED
   emergency department

EDC
   estimated date of confinement

EDI
   electronic data interchange

EEG
   electroencephalogram

effect, placebo
   SEE: placebo effect

effect, side
   SEE: side effect

effect, untoward
   SEE: untoward effect

effective date
   The calendar date on which coverage begins under a health benefit plan.

effectiveness
   The net benefit of a health care technology or service to typical patients in a community practice setting.

efficacy
   The level of benefit expected from a medication, procedure or other medical intervention.

efficiency
   Achieving a desired outcome with the least number of steps or processes.
   SEE: cost-efficiency

EGD
   esophagogastroduodenoscopy

EHL
  electrohydraulic lithotripsy

EIA
  enzyme immunoassay

EKG
  electrocardiogram

elder abuse
  The intentional emotional or physical mistreatment of an aged person.

elder care
  SEE: adult day care

elective
  A procedure, such as surgery, which is not urgent and can be scheduled in advance.

elective admission
  A patient who is hospitalized for a condition that is not urgent, generally scheduled in advance so that appropriate personnel and accommodations are available.

elective surgery
  An operation for a condition that is not immediately life-threatening, and therefore can be scheduled at the convenience of the patient, the physician and other personnel.
  SEE ALSO: emergency surgery

electronic billing
  The input, transmission and submission of third-party claims by way of a computer system.

electronic patient record
  A computerized medical record system that is accessible by providers, payers and other entities involved in the care of a patient.

electrotherapy
  The use of electricity for therapeutic purposes, such as pain relief.

element
1. A unit of datum
2. A primary indicator used as a criterion in an audit.

eligibility, board
> *SEE:* board eligibility

eligibility date
> The calendar date on which an individual is permitted to receive benefits covered by a benefit plan.

eligible
> Having the right to consume health care services covered by a benefit plan.

eligible expenses
> Health care expenses that a benefit plan will accept for coverage.

eligible individual
> *SEE:* beneficiary

eligible person
> *SEE:* beneficiary

elimination period
> A period of time specified in a health benefit contract during which benefits will not be paid.

ELISA
> enzyme-linked immunosorbent assay

ELOS
> estimated length of stay

EM
> emergency medicine

EMCRO
> experimental medical care review organization

emergency
> A serious and unanticipated situation that poses a threat to life or welfare.

emergency admission
A patient admitted to the hospital for the immediate treatment of severe illness or injury that poses a risk of death or disability.
SYN: urgent admission

emergency childbirth
The delivery of a baby that progressed too fast to prepare for standard procedures, such as outside of the hospital.
SYN: precipitate delivery

emergency department (ED, ER)
A hospital outpatient facility that cares for emergent medical and surgical conditions that require immediate attention.
SYN: emergency room

emergency medical services (EMS)
A system of personnel, facilities, communications, equipment and specialized vehicles to care for patients suffering from acute illness or injury. EMS includes an emergency number such as 9-1-1, first responders who provide care at the scene, trained personnel who begin treatment in the field, and hospital facilities and staff equipped to care for emergency situations.
SEE ALSO: emergency department
emergency medical technician
first responder
paramedic
trauma center

emergency medicine
The medical specialty devoted to treatment of acute illness or injury.

emergency physician
A medical doctor who specializes in the diagnosis and treatment of acutely injured or ill patients.

emergency room
SEE: emergency department

emergency surgery
An operation to correct a life-threatening or urgent condition, scheduled at the earliest opportunity.
SEE ALSO: elective surgery

EMG
electromyogram

EMO
exclusive multiple option

employee assistance program (EAP)
Counseling and other services offered to employees on a short-term basis to address mental health or substance abuse issues. Typically refers to other professionals if specialized or longer term care is required.

Employee Retirement Income Security Act (ERISA)
A 1974 federal law that established requirements for self-funded pension and health benefit plans and exempted such plans from state insurance laws.

employer contribution
The portion of the cost of an individual's health benefit paid by the employer.
SEE ALSO: equal-dollar contribution
equal-percentage contribution

employer mandate
A requirement that companies provide health benefit coverage for their employees.

EMS
1. emergency medical services
2. emergency medical systems

EMT
emergency medical technician

EMT-A
emergency medical technician-advanced

encounter
1. One episode of service to a patient.
2. Personal contact between a patient and a physician or other health professional authorized to order diagnostic and treatment services.
   SYN: outpatient visit

encounter data
Information about the health services provided to a patient, used for evaluating the appropriateness and effectiveness of care.

END
endocrinology

endemic
A condition or disease continually found within a population.
SEE ALSO: epidemic
          pandemic

endocrinologist
A physician who specializes in the diagnosis and treatment of diseases affecting the endocrine system.
SEE ALSO: endocrinology

endocrinology
The treatment of diseases involving hormones of the endocrine system, such as diabetes and obesity.

endoscopic surgery
An operative procedure done with the use of tube-like instruments inserted through body orifices or small incisions in the skin that allow visualization and manipulation of internal structures and organs.
SEE ALSO: minimally invasive surgery

endpoint
A measurable factor, such as five-year survival, used to evaluate the outcome of medical care.

ENDT
electroneurodiagnostic technician

enrolled
>   *SEE:* enrollee

enrollee
>   A health maintenance organization member.
>   *SYN:* beneficiary
>   enrolled patient
>   subscriber

enrollment
>   1. The conversion of an eligible group into HMO membership.
>   2. The total number of subscribers in an HMO at a given time.

enrollment area
>   A defined geographic area within which an individual must re-
>   side in order to be eligible to receive health benefit coverage.
>   *SEE ALSO:* out-of-area

enrollment, open
>   *SEE:* open enrollment

enrollment, voluntary
>   *SEE:* voluntary enrollment

en route
>   *SEE:* birth on arrival

ENT
>   ear, nose and throat

entitlement
>   1. Benefits that are mandated by law.
>   2. Traditional benefits that are perceived as rights.

environmental medicine
>   The diagnosis and treatment of allergies, sensitivity, and other
>   illnesses linked to the environment.
>   *SYN:* clinical ecology

EOB
>   explanation of benefits

epidemic
The occurrence of disease at a rate greater than expected within a population within a defined time period.
SEE ALSO: endemic
pandemic

episode, acute
SEE: acute episode

EPO
1. erythropoietin
2. exclusive provider organization

EPSDT
early and periodic screening, diagnosis and treatment

equal-dollar contribution
The portion of health coverage costs paid by the employer, providing a fixed dollar amount regardless of the health plan selected by the employee.

equal-percentage contribution
A portion of health coverage costs paid by the employer, providing the same percentage of the total for each employee regardless of the plan chosen.
SEE ALSO: employer contribution

equivalency, fee-for-service
SEE: fee-for-service equivalency

equivocal
Vague, uncertain or questionable.

ER
emergency room

ERCP
endoscopic retrograde cholangiopancreatography

ERISA
Employee Retirement Income Security Act

ERT
estrogen replacement therapy

escalator clause
A contractual provision that increases the rate of reimbursement for each 12-month period.

ESOP
employee stock ownership program

ESR
erythrocyte sedimentation rate

ESRD
end-stage renal disease

ESWL
extracorporeal shock wave lithotripsy

ET
endotracheal

etiology
The cause of illness or disease.

ETOH
ethyl alcohol

event, qualifying
SEE: qualifying event

event, sentinel
SEE: sentinel event

evidence-based medicine
The treatment of patients based on scientific research rather than tradition or habit.

exacerbation
An increase in the symptoms and severity of an injury or illness.

exception
SEE: waiver

exceptionally large baby
A neonate weighing more than 4,500 grams at birth.

excess capacity
Hospital beds, facilities and staff for which the patient demand no longer exists.

excess-loss
SEE: excess-of-loss
stop-loss

excess-of-loss
A type of insurance purchased by health plans to provide financial coverage above the point where expenses reach a specified level.
SYN: excess-loss
SEE ALSO: stop-loss
stop-loss reinsurance

excess-of-loss insurance
SEE: reinsurance

exclusion
SEE: waiver

exclusions
Specific conditions for which a health benefit plan will not provide coverage.
SYN: exemptions

exclusive dealings clause
SEE: no-shop clause

exclusive provider organization (EPO)
A system of managed care in which providers are paid a discounted fee-for-service rate. Members can choose to receive care by a non-network provider, but usually must pay most or all of the cost.

exclusive remedy
A provision of workers' compensation laws prohibiting lawsuits against employers or co-workers for work-related illness or injury in return for guaranteed first-dollar medical coverage and disability benefits. The workers' compensation system is the exclusive remedy for work-related medical conditions.

exclusivity clause
A contractual provision that prohibits a provider from contracting with another managed care organization.

exemptions
SEE: exclusions

expansion of health resources
Activities that will substantially enhance the type, quality and quantity of health care services.

expected claims
The anticipated level of health care claims from an individual or group during a specific time period.
SEE ALSO: medical break-even point
loss ratio

expenditure, capital
SEE: capital expenditure

expense insurance, surgical
SEE: surgical expense insurance

expenses, accrued
SEE: accrued expenses

expenses, eligible
SEE: eligible expenses

experience, loss
SEE: loss experience

experience period
A specified period of time in which eligible health claims are incurred.
SEE ALSO: incurred claims

experience rating
The calculation of an insurance premium based on the health history of an individual or group.
SEE ALSO: community rating

experience refund
A provision in some benefit plan contracts that returns a portion of premiums to the policyholder if submitted claims are less than anticipated.

expiration date
1. The calendar date on which an insurance policy master contract expires.
2. The calendar date on which an individual is no longer eligible for health benefits.

explanation of benefits
A written statement provided by a third-party payor to the beneficiary after a claim has been reported that indicates the coverage of charges. Charges that are not covered are the responsibility of the patient or another benefit plan.

extended care
Long-term inpatient care in a specialized facility, such as a convalescent or nursing home, usually while recovering after hospitalization.
SYN: convalescent care

extended care facility
A facility that provides long-term skilled nursing care, generally to patients who are recovering after hospitalization.
SYN: convalescent care facility
long-term care facility

extender, physician
SEE: physician assistant

extenders, physician
SEE: physician extenders

extension of benefits
An agreement to maintain eligibility for coverage beyond the scheduled expiration date of a contract, usually limited to a number of days. Typically done to complete treatment begun before the expiration date.

extra risk policy
SEE: rated policy

extracorporeal shock wave lithotripsy
Dissolution of a urinary stone by a device that creates a high-energy shock wave that causes the mineral deposits to crumble or fragment.

extramural birth
A newborn delivered in a non-sterile setting.

extreme immaturity
Describing a neonate with a birth weight of 1,000 grams or less, or a gestational age of 28 complete weeks or less.

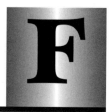

F
fahrenheit

FA
1. first aid
2. functional administration

FACA
Fellow of the American College of Angiology

FACAL
Fellow of the American College of Allergists

FACAn
Fellow of the American College of Anesthesiologists

FACC
Fellow of the American College of Cardiology

FACEP
Fellow, American College of Emergency Physicians

FACG
Fellow of the American College of Gastroenterology

FACHA
Fellow, American College of Hospital Administrators

FACHCA
Fellow of the American College of Health Care Administrators

FACHE
Fellow, American College of Healthcare Executives

facility
One or more buildings, and the equipment and supplies necessary for the delivery of care by health professionals.

facility, ambulatory care
>   *SEE:* ambulatory care facility

facility, domiciliary care
>   *SEE:* residential care facility

facility, extended care
>   *SEE:* extended care facility

facility, institutional-living
>   *SEE:* institutional-living facility

facility, intermediate care
>   *SEE:* intermediate care facility

facility, residential care
>   *SEE:* residential care facility

facility, skilled nursing
>   *SEE:* skilled nursing facility

facility, tertiary care

FACOG
>   Fellow of the American College of Obstetricians and Gynecologists

FACP
>   Fellow of the American College of Physicians

FACPE
>   Fellow, American College of Physician Executives

FACPM
>   Fellow of the American College of Preventive Medicine

FACR
>   Fellow of the American College of Radiology

FACS
>   Fellow of the American College of Surgeons

FACSM
>   Fellow of the American College of Sports Medicine

factor, risk
SEE: risk factor

factor, trend
SEE: trend factor

FAHS
Federation of American Health Systems

fall-out
SEE: disenrollment

fall-out rate
SEE: attrition

family practice
The general medical discipline that addresses routine health needs and the treatment of minor surgical and medical conditions.
SEE ALSO: primary care

family practitioner
A physician who diagnosis and treats uncomplicated medical and surgical conditions, and provides routine health care such as physical examinations and vaccinations.
SEE ALSO: primary care physician

FAS
fetal alcohol syndrome

fasting
1. The purposeful and therapeutic withholding of food, but not water.
2. Referring to a procedure performed on an empty stomach, e.g., "fasting blood sugar."

fatality rate, cause
SEE: cause fatality rate

FBS
fasting blood sugar

FCAP
Fellow of the College of American Pathologists

FCCP
Fellow of the American College of Chest Physicians

FCH
family care home

FDA
Food and Drug Administration

FE
frozen embryo

febrile
Having an elevated temperature.

FEC
free-standing emergency center

federal qualification
The attainment of requirements established by the federal government regulating health maintenance organizations.

federally qualified HMO
A health maintenance organization that meets standards established by the federal government related to corporate structure, health service delivery, provider contracting, quality assurance, financial requirements and grievance procedures.

fee, customary
SEE: customary fee

fee disclosure
The discussion of the charges for health care services by a provider prior to treating a patient.

fee-for-service
A system of reimbursement in which health services are billed and paid separately as they are provided.
SYN: indemnity

fee-for-service, classical
SEE: classical fee-for-service

fee-for-service, discounted
SEE: discounted fee-for-service

fee-for-service equivalency
A comparison between a provider's compensation in an alternate reimbursement system and fee-for-service.

fee-for-service, modified
SEE: modified fee-for-service

fee-for-service, traditional
SEE: traditional fee-for-service

fee, prevailing
SEE: prevailing fee

fee, reasonable
SEE: reasonable fee

fee schedule
A comprehensive list of payment rates for specific procedures or services issued by a managed care company or third-party payer.

fee screen
The determination of customary, prevailing and reasonable charges for physician services by the Health Care Financing Administration, performed at the beginning of each fiscal year.
SYN: prevailing fee

fee splitting
The improper and unethical practice of one physician returning a portion of a referral fee to the physician who made the referral.
SYN: kickback

fee, usual
SEE: usual fee

FFS
fee-for-service

FH
family history

FHR
  fetal heart rate

FI
  fiscal intermediary

FICS
  Fellow of the International College of Surgeons

filter
  A cost-containment mechanism intended to limit utilization of health care resources, such as copayments.

financial consolidation
  The presentation of financial statements of economically integrated but legally separate corporations.
  SEE ALSO: economic consolidation
            economic integration
            financial consolidation

first-dollar coverage
  A health benefit plan which has no deductibles, such as under workers' compensation.

first-generation PPO
  A PPO based on discounted provider fees and limited utilization review.
  SEE ALSO: second-generation PPO
            third-generation PPO

fiscal intermediary (FI)
  An insurance company, administrator, or other entity that accumulates health benefit premiums and distributes payments for health care goods and services. The fiscal intermediary is a third party because it is not directly involved in the delivery of health care.
  SYN: third-party payer

fiscal year (FY)
  A 12-month period used in accounting which may or may not coincide with the calendar year.

fixed costs
Costs that are a function of time rather than volume or level of activity.
SEE ALSO: semivariable costs
variable costs

fixed payment
A premium of a pre-determined value paid for health benefits over a period of time, such as a flat rate per month. Generally used for prospective payment within health maintenance organizations.
SYN: flat rate

flat rate
SEE: fixed payment

fl oz
fluid ounce

flex account
SEE: flexible spending account

flexible spending account (FSA)
An account maintained by an employer that allows individuals to set aside a portion of their salary on a pre-tax basis to pay for out-of-pocket health care costs and child care services. Unlike a medical savings account, money not used at the end of the calendar year may be forfeited.
SYN: flex account

FMB
family maximum benefit

FMC
Foundation for Medical Care

FMG
foreign medical graduate

focused review
A concentrated assessment of a service or department because of high risk, high volume, or an identified problem.

FOP
forensic pathology

formulary
A list of medications that are preferred or required by a managed care company. Physicians may be required to prescribe drugs listed on the formulary under an HMO-physician contract or for prescription drugs to be covered by the health benefit plan.

foundation model
A corporate entity, often a wholly-owned subsidiary of a nonprofit hospital or corporation, that acquires the clinical practices of physicians and contracts for the delivery of medical services to managed care companies and other payers.

FP
family practice

FPP
faculty practice plan

FPS
facial plastic/otolaryngology surgery

FQHMO
federally qualified health maintenance organization

fragmentation
SEE: unbundling

fraternal insurance
A health benefit plan provided to a cooperative group such as a union or social organization for its members.

fraud, claims payment
SEE: claims payment fraud

fraud, claims reporting
SEE: claims reporting fraud

freedom of choice
A health benefit plan provision that allows the eligible person to receive full coverage for care from any licensed provider.

"freedom of choice" law
> *SEE:* any willing provider

freestanding surgical center
> *SEE:* surgicenter

frequency
> The number of times a health care service is provided.

fresh-cell therapy
> *SEE:* live cell therapy

FS
> frozen section

FSA
> flexible spending account

FSOP
> freestanding outpatient facility

FTC
> Federal Trade Commission

FTE
> full-time equivalent

full arrest
> The cessation of respiration and circulation.
> *SEE ALSO:* clinical death

funds, unrestricted
> *SEE:* unrestricted funds

FY
> fiscal year

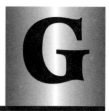

G
gram

gaming the system
Schemes sometimes employed by providers in an attempt to improperly increase the level of compensation from a health care plan, such as inaccurately describing the severity of the patient's condition, the intensity of health services delivered, or rendering care more frequently than medically necessary.
SEE ALSO: code creep
unbundling

GAO
General Accounting Office

gas passer
An informal name for an anesthesiologist.
SEE ALSO: anesthesiologist

gastroenterologist
A physician who specializes in diagnosing and treating conditions of the digestive system.

gastroenterology
The medical specialty related to conditions affecting the digestive system.

gatekeeper
A primary care provider, typically a physician or nurse, to whom a patient is assigned for referral to specialists and access to other health services and facilities. Controls the utilization of services.
SYN: care manager
SEE ALSO: managed care
patient care manager
primary care provider

gatekeeper system
A managed care technique in which patients choose or are assigned a primary care provider who is responsible for controlling referrals to specialists, diagnostic testing and other health services.

GB
governing body

GCR
gross collections revenue

GDP
gross domestic product

GE
gastroenterology

general internal medicine
SEE: internal medicine

generalist
A physician who is not a specialist; one who provides routine health care for minor medical and surgical conditions.

generic screen
The review of medical records using criteria that apply to all patients.

GER
1. geriatric medicine
2. geriatric psychiatry

GERD
gastroesophageal reflux disease

geriatric
Referring to the elderly.

geriatric care management
The coordination of residential and health services for elderly individuals.

geriatric care manager
A professional, often a social worker, who specializes in coordinating the residential and health needs of the elderly.

geriatrician
SEE: gerontologist

geriatrics
SEE: gerontology

gerontologist
A physician who specializes in diagnosing and treating conditions affecting the elderly.
SYN: geriatrician

gerontology
The medical specialty of treating conditions that affect the elderly.
SYN: geriatrics

Gerson therapy
An alternative medicine that employs a nutritional approach to manage chronic and degenerative illnesses.

GH
growth hormone

GHAA
Group Health Association of America
SEE ALSO: American Association of Health Plans

GI
1. gastroenterology
2. gastrointestinal

global budget
1. A limit or cap on total health spending.
2. The national total spent on health care by all payers.
3. A proposed nationwide cap on public and private expenditures for health care services. Price controls or other sanctions would be implemented when specific targets are reached.
SYN: total budget

global pricing

A package pricing of all medical, hospital and physician services related to a specific medical procedure, such as coronary bypass surgery (CABG) or joint replacement. Pricing often includes diagnostic procedures and fees, surgical costs, and post-surgery recovery, rehabilitation and follow-up charges.

SEE ALSO: bundling
package pricing

GME

graduate medical education

GMENAC

Graduate Medical Education National Advisory Committee

GMR

group medical report

GNP

gross national product

GO

gynecological oncology

going bare

An informal term for practicing medicine without having purchased medical malpractice liability insurance.

gomer

A derogatory term for an unpleasant or undesirable patient, an acronym for "get out of my emergency room."

Good Samaritan doctrine

SEE: Good Samaritan law

Good Samaritan law

A law present in some form in many states that provides immunity from liability for volunteers who render emergency first aid in good faith.

SYN: Good Samaritan doctrine
Good Samaritan statute

Good Samaritan statute

SEE: Good Samaritan law

GP
general practice

GPCI
geographic practice cost index

GPM
general preventive medicine

GPP
group practice prepayment plan

GPWW
group practice without walls

gr
grain

graft, cadaver
SEE: cadaver graft

grievance procedures
Mechanisms through which managed care patients can appeal decisions, voice complaints, and obtain relief.

gross
Large; visible to the naked eye.

gross anatomy
The study of structures that can be seen without the aid of a microscope.

gross collections revenue (GCR)
The proportion of gross charges that is collected in cash.

group contract
An agreement between an insurance or health benefit company to provide coverage for a population of persons, such as a group of employees or members of a union.

group, diagnosis-related
SEE: diagnosis-related group

group health insurance
  A health benefit plan in which a large number of individuals are covered under a single contract, such as employees of a company or members of an organization.

group home
  SYN: group-shared housing
  SEE: residential care facility

grouping, peer
  SEE: peer grouping

group model
  A type of health maintenance organization in which the company contracts with one or more medical groups to provide health care services to its membership. The providers remain independent contractors and not employees.

group model HMO
  SEE: closed panel

group, multispecialty
  SEE: multispecialty group

group practice
  A corporation of two or more physicians who maintain an office with shared operating costs and staffing.
  SEE ALSO: limited liability corporation
  professional association
  professional corporation

group practice, prepaid
  SEE: prepaid group practice

group practice without walls (GPWW)
  group practice, medical
  SEE: medical group practice

group-shared housing
  SEE: group home

GS
  general surgery

gt
drop

gtt
drops

GTT
glucose tolerance test

guaranteed issue
1. A legal or regulatory requirement that health insurance carriers accept all who apply for coverage.
2. A provision in an employer's health benefit plan that allows automatic acceptance and coverage of any employee of the company.

guideline, treatment
SEE: treatment protocol

GVS
general vascular surgery

GY
graduate year

GYN
gynecology

gynecologist
A physician who specializes in the diagnosis and treatment of conditions affecting the female reproductive system.

gynecology
The medical specialty related to the diagnosis and treatment of disorders of the female reproductive system.

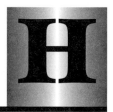

h
> hour

HAA
> Hospice Association of America

HAD
> health care alternatives development

HBV
> Hepatitis B virus

HCFA
> Health Care Financing Administration

HCO
> health care organization

HCPOTP
> health care providers other than physicians

HCQIA
> Health Care Quality Improvement Act

HCT
> hematocrit

health
> 1. A state absent of disease and of maximal well-being.
> 2. A state of complete physical, mental and social well-being, and not merely the absence of disease or infirmity.

health agency, home
> *SEE:* home health agency

health alliance
> *SEE:* alliance

health care, catastrophic
SEE: catastrophic health care

health care, community-based
SEE: community-based health care

health care consumer
SEE: patient

health care, home
SEE: home health care

health care, hospital-based
SEE: hospital-based health care

health care proxy
A legal document designating a person authorized to make health care decisions on behalf of another in the event the patient's decision-making abilities are incapacitated.
SEE ALSO: durable power of attorney

health care service
Activities that contribute to the physical, mental and social well-being of patients.
SEE ALSO: medical services
nursing services

health care staff
Licensed professionals, such as physicians and nurses, who are responsible for patient care within an organization or facility.
SEE ALSO: allied health personnel
physician extenders

health care support services
Activities that enable the delivery of medical care within an organization, but not directly involved in patient care. Support services include medical records, housekeeping, medical transcription and paging.

health care system
An organization of hospitals and health care-related entities linked by ownership, management contracts, or other corporate arrangements.

Syn: network
See also: horizontal integration
vertical integration

health insurance adjuster
See: adjuster

health insurance, group
See: group health insurance

health insurance, substandard
See: substandard health insurance

health insurance, supplemental
See: supplemental health insurance

health maintenance organization (HMO)
A system of health care services in which providers accept a prospective payment at a capitated rate per patient rather than fee-for-service. Patients are assigned a gatekeeper from a closed panel of physicians who provides primary care and referral to specialists. This system has low deductibles and co-payments, and severe reduction in benefits for self-referral or out-of-network services.
See also: capitation
closed panel
gatekeeper
group model HMO
independent practice association
network model HMO
prospective payment
staff model HMO

health maintenance organization, social
See: social health maintenance organization

Health Plan Employer Data and Information Set (HEDIS)
A set of uniform, standardized performance measures employed for comparison among health benefit plans.

health plan purchasing cooperative (HPPC)
A proposed regional organization that acts as an agent for group of employers in the purchase of health care services. By pooling smaller groups into a large collective, the HPPC can use economies of scale to negotiate better prices with providers.

health resources, expansion of
SEE: expansion of health resources

health screening
A process of evaluating the pre-existing conditions and health risks of applicants with the intent of identifying those who are likely to produce high health care costs.

health service area
A defined geographic area served by a program or facility.
SYN: catchment area
service area

health services, supplemental
SEE: supplemental health services

health system
A corporate organization comprised of at least one hospital and a group of physicians.

health, community
SEE: community health

HEDIS
Health Plan Employer Data Information Set

HEENT
head, eyes, ears, nose and throat

HEM
hematology

hematologist
A physician who specializes in the diagnosis and treatment of blood disorders.

hematology
The treatment of blood disorders.

hemiplegia
Paralysis of one side of the body, usually due to trauma or disease of the brain or spinal cord.

herbal medicine
An alternative medicine employing the therapeutic use of botanical, herbs or other plant material.

herbalism
SEE: herbal medicine

hesitation payment
SEE: token payment

Hgb
hemoglobin

HH
home health services

HHA
home health agency

HHS
Health and Human Services

HI
1. horizontal integration
2. hospital insurance

HIAA
Health Insurance Association of America

HIB
haemophilus influenza b

high index of suspicion
A principle of medical care that encourages providers to think in terms of worst-case scenarios. When confronted with several possible causes of the patient's signs and symptoms, the physician should consider and rule out the most serious and consequential diagnoses first. For example, a victim of a car crash should be treated as though there is a fracture of the neck or spine until it can be proven otherwise by x-rays and evaluation.
SEE ALSO: index of suspicion

HIN
hospital insurance network

HIO
health insuring organization

HIPC
health insurance purchasing cooperative

HIS
hospital information system

HISB
health insurance standards board

histologic technician
An individual who works under the supervision of a pathologist or other medical director and assists with the preparation of specimens for examination.

histologic technologist
SEE: histotechnologist

histologist
A physician who specializes in the study of cells, tissue and organs.

histology
The study of the structure and function of cells, tissue and organs.

histopathologist
A physician, often a pathologist, who specializes in the study of abnormal or diseased cells, tissues or organs.
SEE ALSO: pathologic histologist

histopathology
The study of the structure and function of diseased or abnormal cells, tissue or organs.
SYN: pathologic histology

histopathology laboratory
A special unit in a hospital or other medical facility in which diseased or abnormal cells, tissue or organs are prepared and studied.

history
> The portion of the physical examination in which the provider elicits information about the nature of the patient's condition, such as its course in the past. Also pertinent to the history is the presence of similar or related conditions among the patient's family members.

histotechnologist
> A licensed or certified professional with at least a baccalaureate degree who studies diseased cells, tissue or organs. Works under the supervision of a pathologist or other medical director. May supervise histologic technicians.
>
> *SYN:* histologic technologist

HIV
> human immunodeficiency virus

HMD
> hyaline membrane disease

HMO
> health maintenance organization

HMO, federally qualified
> *SEE:* federally qualified HMO

HMSA
> health manpower shortage area

HNS
> head and neck surgery

HOI
> Health Outcomes Institute

hold harmless
> A clause in a contract relieving the payer of potential liability that may arise from the delivery of health care.

holism
> *SEE:* holistic medicine

holistic medicine

A philosophy that recognizes the physical, emotional, and mental aspects of the individual and encourages seeing patients as a whole person rather than a disease or set of symptoms. Typically emphasizes prevention and greater involvement of the patient in health care.

SYN: holism

home care

A program to provide health and psychosocial services in the patient's home, with the goal of maintaining the patient's wellbeing and avoiding hospitalization.

home for the aged

SEE: nursing home

home health agency (HHA)

A public or private organization that provides medical and nursing services to patients at their place of residence.

home health agency, Medicare-certified

SEE: Medicare-certified home health agency

home health care

The delivery of medical and nursing services in a residential or noninstitutional setting, often the home of the patient or relative.

SYN: home health service

home health service

SEE: home health care

home visit

Care provided in a patient's residence.

SYN: house call

homograft

Transplantation of tissue taken from the patient, such as using harvested skin to cover a burn.

horizontal integration

The organization of similar groups of providers, generally in different geographic markets.

SEE ALSO: vertical integration

hospice
A multidisciplinary program providing health, psychological, and social services to terminally ill patients and their families.

hospice care
Health services provided to terminally ill patients and their families.

hospital
A health care facility with inpatient beds, a medical and nursing staff available 24 hours a day, ancillary services, and often medical and surgical services, such as ambulatory care and home health care.
SEE ALSO: community hospital
            health care facility
            tertiary care

hospital affiliation
1. A contractual arrangement by which a hospital provides inpatient care for members of a health maintenance organization.
2. An inpatient facility where a physician has admitting privileges.

hospital-based health care services
Patient care delivered through an inpatient medical facility, such as home health care, ambulatory care, and rehabilitation.
SEE ALSO: community-based health care services

hospital-based services

hospital boarder
A person lodged at a hospital who is not a patient, such as a person waiting for next-day surgery or a family member who sleeps at the hospital to be near the patient.
SYN: boarder

hospital, community
SEE: community hospital

hospital expense insurance
An insurance policy that covers the costs of hospitalization in the event of illness or injury.

hospital indemnity
An insurance policy that pays a specified amount of money directly to the beneficiary on a daily, weekly or monthly basis in the event of hospitalization. The compensation is not related to the costs of medical care and is not restricted to any purposes.

hospital inpatient
A person who receives medical care while admitted for at least one overnight stay in a hospital.

hospitalization
Admission to an inpatient facility for one or more nights.

hospitalization, average duration of
SEE: average duration of hospitalization

hospitalization, duration of inpatient
SEE: length of stay

hospitalization, partial
SEE: partial hospitalization

hospital newborn inpatient
An infant patient admitted after birth in the hospital, as opposed to birth outside of the hospital or transferred from another facility.

hospital outpatient
A patient who occupies a hospital bed but is not admitted for an overnight stay. The patient may be treated in an outpatient facility or be under observation.
SEE ALSO: observation patient
short-stay patient

hospital patient
A person who receives health care services from a hospital, either as an inpatient admitted for an overnight stay or through affiliated programs, facilities or services.

hospital, swing-bed
SEE: swing-bed hospital

hospital, teaching
SEE: teaching hospital

hospital, voluntary
> SEE: voluntary hospital

hospital, weekend
> SEE: weekend hospital

house call
> SEE: home visit

house staff
> Medical students and residents affiliated with a teaching hospital.

housing, group-shared
> SEE: group home

housing, matched
> SEE: matched housing

Hoxey therapy
> An unproven cancer therapy involving specially formulated herbal tonics and a strict dietary regimen.

H&P
> history and physical

HPA
> hospital-physician alliance

HPI
> history of present illness

HPO
> hospital-physician organization

HPPC
> health plan purchasing cooperative

HPSA
> health professional shortage area

HPV
> human papilloma virus

HR
> 1. House resolution
> 2. human resources

HRA
1. health records analyst
2. health risk assessment

HRF
health-related facility

HRSA
Health Resources and Services Administration

HRT
hormone replacement therapy

h.s.
hour of sleep; at bedtime

HS
hand surgery

HSA
1. health services agency
2. health services agreement
3. health systems agency

HSB
health standards board

HSM
hospital, surgical, and medical benefits

HSP
health systems plan

HSV-1
herpes simplex virus Type 1

HSV-2
herpes simplex virus Type 2

Ht
height

HTN
hypertension

HX
> history

hybrid managed care
> A managed health care plan with point-of-service provisions that allow patients to choose out-of-network providers, usually by bearing a greater share of the cost.
> *SEE ALSO:* open-ended HMO
> point-of-service

hydrogen peroxide therapy
> An alternative medicine employing the injection of hydrogen peroxide for claimed beneficial effects.

hydrotherapy
> The use of water for therapeutic effects.

hyperbaric therapy
> The use of a pressurized chamber to treat medical conditions, such as smoke inhalation, gangrene or diving injury.

hypnotherapy
> The use of hypnosis for therapeutic purposes, such as the treatment of addiction.

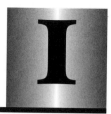

IAF
industry adjustment factor

iatrogenic disease
An illness, injury, infection or complication resulting from medical care. Causes of iatrogenic disease include diagnostic procedures, treatment, surgery, medication or sub-optimal patient care.
SEE ALSO: nosocomial disease

IBNR
incurred but not reported

ICD
1. implantable cardioverter defibrillator
2. International Classification of Diseases

ICF
intermediate care facility

ICMA
Individual Case Management Association

ICU
intensive care unit

I&D
incision and drainage

ID
1. infectious disease
2. intradermal

IDDM
insulin-dependent diabetes mellitus

identification, personal
> *SEE:* personal identification

idiopathic
> of unknown origin

IDS
> integrated delivery system

IG
> immunology

IHN
> integrated health network

IHS
> integrated health system

illness, acute
> *SEE:* acute illness

illness, severity of
> *SEE:* severity of illness

IM
> 1. internal medicine
> 2. intramuscular

imagery
> The use of mental images or symbols affect change on a physical or psychological condition.
> *SYN:* directed imagery
> guided imagery
> visualization

immaturity, extreme
> *SEE:* extreme immaturity

immobility
> The restriction of a patient's ability to move.

immobilization
> The act of rendering a patient unable to move part or all of the body.

immunity
1. The biological resistance to infectious disease.
2. An exemption to legal liability.

immunologist
A physician who specializes in the diagnosis and treatment of allergies and infectious disease.

immunology
The study of allergies and the body's response to infectious agents and other disease.

IMP
impression

implant
The surgical grafting or insertion of material into body tissue.

implied consent
Permission that is not explicitly written or spoken, but can be inferred by behavior or inaction that leads one to believe that consent has been given. For example, the act of rolling up the sleeve implies that the patient consents to having blood drawn.
  SEE ALSO: imposed consent

imposed consent
The involuntary submission to testing or treatment that is required by law, such as drug or alcohol testing, vaccination or screening for sexually transmitted disease.

in-home care
Assistance with activities of daily living, housekeeping and other nursing services provided in the patient's home. Intended to postpone the need for hospitalization.
  SYN: home health care

in-service volunteer
A person who works in a regular, responsible position in a health care facility, but does not get paid for their time and does not replace paid personnel.

incentive
A reward, usually financial, for following a desired pattern of behavior.

incentive program
A health benefit program which pays providers an increasing percentage of the cost of treatment if prescribed patient care guidelines are followed.

incidence
The number of new cases of a disease occurring within a defined population during a specific period of time.
SEE ALSO: prevalence

incidental procedure
A procedure associated with a professional service, but not the primary purpose of the patient visit, such as measuring the blood pressure.

incontinence
The inability to control the bladder, the bowel or both.

incremental cost
SEE: marginal cost

incubation period
The period of time between infection with a disease-producing agent and the onset of symptoms.
SYN: prodromal period

incurred but not reported (IBNR)
Health care claims known or suspected to have been incurred within a specified time period but not reported to the insurer; an estimation of a health plan's financial liability.

incurred claims
The actual liability for reported and covered health care costs within a specified past time period.
SEE ALSO: experience period
loss experience
medical loss ratio

incurred claims loss ratio
The liability for claims that are incurred, paid and unpaid, during a specified time period, divided by premiums.
SEE ALSO: loss ratio

IND
Investigational new drug

indemnification schedule
SEE: table of allowances

indemnity
An insurance policy that provides reimbursement for financial loss, or in the case of health insurance, pays for medical goods and services.

indemnity benefits
Insurance benefits paid directly in cash to the beneficiary, rather than paying for services.
SYN: indemnity insurance
SEE ALSO: service benefits

indemnity carrier
An insurance company or non-profit organization that provides coverage for individuals or groups of people according to a contract that specifies premiums, benefits and exclusions.
SYN: insurer

indemnity, double
SEE: accidental death benefit

indemnity, hospital
SEE: hospital indemnity

indemnity insurance
SEE: indemnity benefits

indemnity, managed
SEE: managed indemnity

indemnity plan
A health benefit plan in which a third party pays a specific amount for health care services and goods, regardless of actual charges. Benefits may be paid to the provider by assignment, or directly to the beneficiary.
SEE ALSO: assignment of benefits
direct reimbursement

independent practice association (IPA)
A model of health maintenance organization in which providers own and maintain independent offices. Providers are contracted with managed care companies for services at discounted or capitated rates, though they are usually allowed to accept fee-for-service patients as well.

index of suspicion
An approach to diagnosis demanding that the most serious possible disease or injury states be identified and ruled out first.

indicator
A measure of health care quality and appropriateness based on clinically valid and reliable factors.
SYN: screen

indigent, medically
SEE: medically indigent

individual insurance
A health benefit policy sold directly through a carrier to an individual, rather than as a member of a larger group. Typically more extensive than group health insurance.
SYN: individual policy
SEE ALSO: group health insurance
non-group insurance
personal insurance

individual policy
SEE: individual insurance

industrial screening
A process by which new employees are systematically put through a battery of medical tests to identify risk factors and susceptibility to disease or injury at the worksite prior to job placement.

infant, post-term
SEE: post-term infant

infant, preterm
SEE: preterm infant

infection, nosocomial
SEE: nosocomial disease

information, release of
SEE: release of information

injury
1. Physical damage to the body resulting from a wound or trauma.
2. An illness, disease or other harm, physical or economic, that is a subject of a medical malpractice liability action or claim.
SYN: trauma

injury, non-disabling
SEE: non-disabling injury

inpatient
1. A person admitted for an overnight stay in a hospital.
2. Referring to medical services provided during hospitalization.

inpatient bed count day
The number of beds available in a health care facility during a 24-hour period.
SEE ALSO: bed count

inpatient care
Medical services provided to a person admitted for an overnight stay in a hospital.
SEE ALSO: outpatient care

inpatient census
The actual number of inpatient patients receiving care in a hospital during a specified time period.

inpatient day
SEE: inpatient services day

inpatient days of stay
SEE: length of stay

inpatient, hospital
SEE: hospital inpatient

inpatient, hospital newborn
SEE: hospital newborn inpatient

inpatient services day
The health care services received by a patient in a 24-hour period.
SYN: bed occupancy day
census day
inpatient day
patient day
resident day

insolvency plan
Provisions, such as insurance, to maintain health care benefits in the event an HMO becomes insolvent. Required of federally qualified HMOs.

institutional review board (IRB)
An academic medical center committee designated to review and approve research involving human volunteer subjects, as required by federal regulations.

insurance
A written contract that protects an individual or company against the financial risks of events that may occur in the future.

insurance, business
    SEE: business insurance

insurance company
    A corporation whose primary purpose is to issue contracts to groups and individuals that assume risk for future financial losses.
    SYN: carrier
           insurer

insurance company, mutual
    SEE: mutual insurance company

insurance company, stock
    SEE: stock insurance company

insurance, comprehensive major medical
    SEE: comprehensive major medical insurance

insurance, dread disease
    SEE: dread disease insurance

insurance, fraternal
    SEE: fraternal insurance

insurance, group health
    SEE: group health insurance

insurance, health
    SEE: health insurance

insurance, hospital expense
    SEE: hospital expense insurance

insurance, individual
    SEE: individual insurance

insurance, mail order
    SEE: mail order insurance

insurance, malpractice
    SEE: malpractice insurance

insurance, MediGap
    SEE: Medicare supplemental policy

insurance, professional liability
> *SEE:* professional liability insurance

insurance, substandard health
> *SEE:* substandard health insurance

insurance, supplemental health
> *SEE:* supplemental health insurance

insurance, surgical expense
> *SEE:* surgical expense insurance

insurance, workers' compensation
> *SEE:* workers' compensation insurance

insured
> *SEE:* beneficiary
> member

insurer
> *SEE:* insurance company

integrated delivery system (IDS)
> An organization of providers to enhance cost-efficiency and co-ordinate care by hospitals and physicians. May include a component to finance as well as deliver health care.
> *SEE ALSO:* integrated provider network
> integrated system
> integration

integrated provider network (IPN)
> An organization of primary and specialized physicians, hospitals and other providers operating within a defined geographic area who contract as a single unit to provide care to defined patient populations.

integrated system
> An organization including at least one hospital, a network of physicians and other providers, along with ancillary services, outpatient diagnostic and treatment facilities, that offers a comprehensive range of health care services.

integration
The development of organizational relationships, through ownership or contract, among hospitals, physicians and other providers to enhance cost-effectiveness and patient care. Integration often involves the meshing of a health maintenance organization (HMO) with the medical services providers in an integrated system.
SEE ALSO: clinical integration
economic integration
horizontal integration
vertical integration

integration, clinical
SEE: clinical integration

integration, economic
SEE: economic integration

integration, horizontal
SEE: horizontal integration

integration, vertical
SEE: vertical integration

inter-hospital transfer
The movement of a patient from one health facility to another, typically by ambulance.

interdisciplinary
Employing the expertise of more than one specialized area.

interdisciplinary audit
An evaluation of patient care involving professionals or allied personnel from two or more medical specialties.

intermediary
An insurance company authorized by the Health Care Financing Administration to process Medicare Part A claims.

intermediary, fiscal
SEE: fiscal intermediary

intermediate care facility
An inpatient facility that provides health care for patients who do not require the level of care of a skilled nursing facility or hospital.

intermediate outcome
The status of a patient at a designated point during the course of treatment and recovery.

internal medicine
The general medical discipline involved in the diagnosis and treatment of disorders of the internal organs in adult patients.
SYN: general internal medicine

internist
A generalist physician who diagnoses and treats conditions affecting the internal organs.

intradermal
Within the skin; a means of administering medications by injection.

intramuscular (IM)
Into the muscle; a method of administering medications.

intravenous (IV)
By way of a vein, a method of administering fluids or medications to a patient.

invasive
Describing a diagnostic or therapeutic procedure involving the insertion of a device or instrument through the skin or body orifice. Usually refers to surgery.
SEE ALSO: minimally invasive surgery
noninvasive

investigational new drug (IND)
A medication that is not yet approved by the Food and Drug Administration for routine use and is available for experimental use only, generally to evaluate efficacy and safety.

IOL
intraocular lens implant

IP
1. immunopathology
2. inpatient

IPA
independent practice association

IPN
integrated provider network

IRB
institutional review board

iridology
A philosophy of alternative medicine in which the iris is studied to diagnose disease.

ISHA
International Subacute Healthcare Association

isolation
The separation of a patient from others by containment and the use of barriers in order to prevent the spread of disease and protect the patient.

issue, guaranteed
SEE: guaranteed issue

IUD
intrauterine device

IV
Intravenous; a route for the administration of fluids or medication.

IVP
intravenous pyelogram

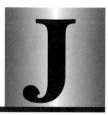

JCAHO

Joint Commission for the Accreditation of Healthcare Organizations

job lock

An informal term for the reluctance to change one's employment situation because of concern about losing or changing health benefits.

joint study committee

An advisory group comprised of representatives from two or more organizations that makes recommendations about proposed mergers or collaborative efforts.

joint venture

A business undertaking by two or more entities in which the parties share resources and risk, but otherwise remain independent. Often involves investment in equity ownership by some or all participating parties.

JPA

joint powers authority

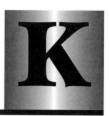

kg
kilogram

kickback
SEE: fee splitting

KUB
kidney, ureter, bladder

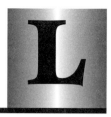

L
1. left
2. liter

Laban movement analysis
A system for observing and interpreting movement, often used in conjunction with dance therapy.

laboratory diagnosis
The determination of the nature of a disease by chemical, microscopic, microbiologic, immunologic or pathologic study of the patient's tissue or body fluids.

laboratory, histopathology
SEE: histopathology laboratory

lap chole
Laparoscopic cholecystectomy; the minimally invasive removal of the gallbladder.
SYN: lap choly
SEE ALSO: minimally invasive surgery

lap choly
SEE: lap chole

laparoscopic surgery
An operative procedure in which internal structures are visualized and manipulated by an optical instrument passed through small incisions in the skin.
SYN: minimally invasive surgery
SEE ALSO: open surgery

LAR
laryngology

large case management
>SEE: catastrophic case management

lb
>pound

LCAH
>life care at home

LCM
>large case management

learning disability
>A disorder involving the understanding or use of language, which may impair the ability to read, write, speak, or perform calculations.

least expensive alternative treatment (LEAT)
>A provision in a health benefit plan that permits coverage for the least costly procedure when more than one treatment option exists.
>>SYN: least expensive professionally acceptable alternative treatment (LEPAAT)

least expensive professionally acceptable alternative treatment (LEPAAT)
>SEE: least expensive alternative treatment

LEAT
>least expensive alternative treatment

LEEP
>loop electrosurgical excision procedure

length of stay (LOS)
>The number of days a patient is hospitalized, or in a unit of the hospital (i.e., intensive care), per episode of illness or injury.
>>SYN: days of stay
>>discharge days
>>duration of inpatient hospitalization
>>inpatient days of stay

LEPAAT
Least expensive professionally acceptable alternative treatment

LH
luteinizing hormone

liability
An obligation, often financial, that one is legally bound to fulfill.

licensure
Authority granted by the state for an individual to perform a trade or business that would otherwise be unlawful.
SEE ALSO: certification
registration

life care at home
A comprehensive package of health services provided by a single agency that allows patients to remain at home while assured access to health care facilities. Typically includes housekeeping assistance, meals, admission to assisted living and hospital facility, and emergency responses.
SYN: life care without walls

life care without walls
SEE: life care at home

life extension
Endeavors to enhance life expectancy, such as drugs, nutritional supplements, diets and other forms of alternative medicine.

lifetime aggregate
The maximum benefit provided for major medical conditions.

lifetime disability benefit
Payments to an individual for as long as he or she is disabled, even if that is the remainder of the person's life.
SYN: long-term disability income insurance
SEE ALSO: disability benefit

limit, stop-loss
SEE: stop-loss limit

limitation, benefit
    SEE: benefit limitation

limitations
    Conditions in a health benefit contract that restrict health benefit coverage, such as waiting periods or limits on the extent of certain health services.
    SYN: restrictions
    SEE ALSO: exclusions

limited liability company (LLC)
    A hybrid form of business often used by small companies, such as medical practices, that combines the legal protection of incorporation with the tax advantages of a partnership.

limited policy
    A health insurance contract only covering specific conditions or injuries.

limited-stay patient
    SEE: short-stay patient

liquidity
    The ability to pay debts as they become due.

list, waiting
    SEE: waiting list

lithotripsy
    The crushing of a stone in the kidney, bladder or ureter.
    SEE ALSO: extracorporeal shock wave lithotripsy

lithotripsy, extracorporeal shock wave
    SEE: extracorporeal shock wave lithotripsy

live birth
    The delivery of an infant that shows evidence of life, such as a heartbeat or respiration, regardless of the duration of pregnancy.

live cell therapy
    The administration of fetal animal cells for therapeutic benefits.
    SYN: cellular therapy
           fresh-cell therapy

live-in unit
A room or other facility maintained by a hospital for use by parents while their children are hospitalized.

lives, covered
SEE: covered lives

living will
An advance directive expressing a person's wishes regarding life-sustaining care in the event he or she becomes incompetent. Typically, the living will directs the physician to withhold treatments or procedures that prolong the dying process and are not necessary for comfort.
SYN: terminal care document
SEE ALSO: advance directive

Livingston treatment
An unproven remedy claimed to enhance the body's immune system, emphasizing a diet of raw vegetables.

LLC
limited liability corporation

LLQ
left lower quadrant

LM
legal medicine

load
The portion of the price of an insurance policy that is accounted by the cost of acquisition, profit, reserves and other administrative expenses.

load, administrative
SEE: administrative load

load, risk
SEE: risk adjustment

loading, administrative
SEE: administrative loading

LOB
line of business

LOC
loss of consciousness

localized
Referring to a condition that is limited to a defined area or part of the body.
SEE ALSO: systemic

lock-in
A requirement that all medical services received by the members of a managed care plan be provided or authorized by the plan or its physicians. Exceptions are usually made for medical emergencies, and urgent health needs that occur while the patient is temporarily outside a managed care plan's service area.

long-term care
Health care services provided in a non-acute care facility to a resident or patient with a condition that does not require continual supervision and assistance by health care professionals in an acute care facility.

long-term care facility
SEE: extended care facility

long-term disability (LTD)
Partial or permanent incapacitation as a result of illness or injury lasting more than three to six months.
SEE ALSO: partial disability
temporary disability
total disability

long-term disability income insurance
SEE: lifetime disability benefit

LOS
length of stay

loss experience
Total incurred claims, paid claims, and estimated incurred but not reported (IBNR) under an insured or self-insured benefit plan.
SEE ALSO: incurred but not reported
incurred claims
loss ratio

loss of income benefits
SEE: disability benefits

loss ratio
The sum of paid claims, incurred claims and expenses divided by premium revenues received during a specified time period.
SEE ALSO: break-even point
incurred but not reported
loss experience
medical loss ratio

loss ratio, incurred claims
SEE: incurred claims loss ratio

loss ratio, paid claims
SEE: paid claims loss ratio

low birth weight neonate
A newborn whose birth weight is 2,500 grams or less, regardless of gestational age.

low-volume DRGs
Categories of diagnosis related groups (DRGs) in which a hospital has five or fewer cases in its base year.

LP
lumbar puncture

LPN
licensed practical nurse

LTC
long-term care

LTD
  long-term disability

LTP
  laryngotracheobronchitis

lumbar puncture (LP)
  The insertion of a needle into the spinal canal to obtain fluid for diagnosis or therapeutic purposes.
  SYN: spinal tap

lump sum settlement
  Resolution of a debt in one large payment rather than smaller amounts over a period of time.

LUQ
  left upper quadrant

L&W
  living and well

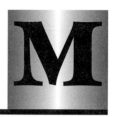

m
meter

MAA
medical assistance for the aged

MAC
maximum allowable cost

magnetic therapy
The use of magnets or magnetic fields for therapeutic effects.

mail order insurance
Life, health or disability insurance policies typically sold by direct mail or mass advertising. Typically requires no physician examination, has relatively high premiums and low rate of claims recovery.

maintenance drug therapy
The reduction of a drug dose to the lowest level that achieves the desired therapeutic effect.

major diagnosis
The patient's condition that requires most resources during hospitalization. May be different than the admitting diagnosis.

major diagnostic categories (MDCs)
A system for classifying patients into medically meaningful groupings.
SEE ALSO: diagnosis-related groups
ambulatory surgery categories

major medical
SEE: catastrophic coverage

major medical insurance, comprehensive
SEE: comprehensive major medical insurance

malignant
Referring to a condition that is harmful or cancerous.

malpractice insurance
SEE: professional liability insurance

managed care
An integrated system of delivering and financing health services, the purpose of which is to ensure that care is appropriate and cost-effective, and of high quality. Managed care emphasizes primary care and restricts utilization of specialty care, costly procedures, and hospitalization by means of utilization review and utilization management processes. Often employs a primary care physician, usually called a gatekeeper, to control referrals to specialists. May also feature a network of selected providers who are contracted for comprehensive health services; a process of credentialing health care providers; formal quality assurance and utilization review programs; a benefit design that gives patients a financial incentive to choose services from in-network providers.
  SEE ALSO: exclusive provider organization
                 fee-for-service
                 health maintenance organization
                 preferred provider organization
                 quality assurance
                 utilization review

managed care, hybrid
SEE: hybrid managed care

managed care organization (MCO)
An organization that provides managed health care, such as a health maintenance organization (HMO), a preferred provider organization (PPO), or exclusive provider organization (EPO).
  SEE ALSO: managed care

managed competition
A model of health care financing and delivery proposed by the Jackson Hole Group in which insurers and health maintenance organizations (HMOs) offer standard benefit packages, with optional additional coverage, and compete in the marketplace

based on price. In theory, by limiting tax deductions for health care expenses and charging more for liberal benefit plans, consumer demand for affordable coverage would slow the growth of health care costs.

managed indemnity
A form of traditional indemnity health benefits that employ limited mechanisms to control utilization and/or cost of care.
SEE ALSO: managed care

management, catchment area
SEE: catchment area management

management, disease
SEE: disease management

management, geriatric care
SEE: geriatric care management

management, outcomes
SEE: outcomes management

management services organization (MSO)
A company, usually a wholly owned subsidiary of a non-profit hospital or corporation, that manages support services for physician practices and contracts for health care services with managed care companies and other payers. Some MSOs are publicly held or private corporations that manage many physician practices.

management, utilization
SEE: utilization management

manager, claims
SEE: claims manager

manager, clinic
SEE: clinic manager

manager, unit
SEE: unit manager

manager, ward
SEE: unit manager

mandate
A requirement established by law. For example a federal law requiring that companies offer employees access to an HMO that properly bids on the business if 25 or more workers live within the HMO service area.

mandated benefits
Health care coverage required to be offered by state or federal law.

mandated employer insurance
    SEE: employer mandate

MAP
1. maximum allowable cost
2. mean arterial pressure

marginal cost
The incremental cost of providing an additional unit of a health care service or product, with the original investment costs factored out.
    SYN: differential cost
            incremental cost

marked
Significant or noteworthy.

market power
    SEE: market share

market share
The percentage of the total market captured by a health maintenance organization or other health benefit plan.
    SYN: market power
    SEE ALSO: penetration

massage therapy
The manipulation of skin and muscle for therapeutic purposes.

mastectomy
Surgical removal of the breast.
    SEE ALSO: lumpectomy

matched housing
> *SEE:* shared housing

maximum allowable
> *SEE:* allowed amount

maximum allowable charges
> The maximum dollar amount specified in a health plan contract that is payable toward the cost of covered health care services.
> *SYN:* maximum allowance
> *SEE ALSO:* allowed amount

maximum allowance
> *SEE:* maximum allowable charges

maximum, benefit
> *SEE:* benefit maximum

MCE
Medical care evaluation

MCH
mean corpuscular hemoglobin

MCHC
mean corpuscular hemoglobin concentration

MCM
1. medical case management
2. Medicare carriers manual

MCO
managed care organization

MCP
managed care plan

MCV
mean corpuscular volume

MD
1. manic-depressive
2. medical director
3. medical doctor
4. muscular dystrophy

MDC
major diagnostic categories

ME
1. medical education
2. medical examiner

measurable
Having characteristics to be objectively assessed for the purposes of comparison.

measure
A device, such as a statistic, for assessing the quality or quantity of health care service.

measure, outcome
SEE: outcome measure

measure, performance
SEE: performance measure

measure, risk
SEE: risk measure

Medicaid
A joint federal-state program to provide health insurance to low-income families and nursing home services to low-income elderly persons.

medical advice, against
SEE: against medical advice

medical doctor
SEE: physician

medical equipment, durable
SEE: durable medical equipment

medical expense reimbursement plan
SEE: noncontributory plan

medical foundation
SEE: foundation model

medical group, participating
> *SEE:* participating medical group

medical group practice
> The delivery of health services by three or more physicians through a formally organized entity that provides equipment, personnel, information systems and business management.

medical IRA
> *SEE:* medical savings account

medical loss ratio (MLR)
> The total of losses—paid, unpaid, and incurred but not reported —for medical, hospital and physician services incurred by an insurer, a health maintenance organization (HMO) or other prepaid health plan, divided by the amount of premiums or revenue collected.
> *SEE ALSO:* incurred but not reported
> loss experience
> loss ratio

medical practice plan
> *SEE:* treatment protocol

medical savings account (MSA)
> A proposed system by which individuals would be permitted to set aside money on a pre-tax basis to pay for health care costs. Unlike a flex account, the amount set aside in a medical savings account is not lost at the end of the calendar year.
> *SYN:* medical IRA

medical services, emergency
> *SEE:* emergency medical services

medical social work
> The coordination between social services and patients who require these services to address medical issues. Medical social workers also often help patients and families adjust to living with illness and obtain maximum health care benefits.

medical staff, chief of
> *SEE:* chief of staff

medically indigent
A person lacking sufficient insurance coverage, income, or resources to pay the full cost of health care.
SYN: underinsurance
uninsured

medically induced disease
SEE: iatrogenic disease

medically necessary
Describing a treatment or service determined to be required to establish or maintain the health of a patient, based on the prevailing standards of care in the professional community and the clinical judgment of the provider.

Medicare
A federal program that provides health insurance benefits for the disabled and for people 65 years of age and older.

Medicare-certified home health agency
A home health agency that is authorized to receive reimbursement for services provided to Medicare beneficiaries.

Medicare Part A
A program that provides the elderly benefits for hospitalization, home health care, hospice, and skilled nursing facility services.

Medicare Part B
A program that provides the elderly with benefits that cover physician services, medical supplies, and other outpatient care.

Medicare supplemental policy
SEE: Medigap

medicine, bariatric
SEE: bariatric medicine

medicine, botanical
SEE: herbal medicine

medicine, cookbook
SEE: cookbook medicine

medicine, emergency
    SEE: emergency medicine

medicine, environmental
    SEE: environmental medicine

medicine, evidence-based
    SEE: evidence-based medicine

medicine, holistic
    SEE: holistic medicine

medicine, internal
    SEE: internal medicine

medicine, nuclear
    SEE: nuclear medicine

medicine, podiatric
    SEE: podiatry

medicine, preventive
    SEE: preventive medicine

Medigap
    A supplemental private insurance policy to cover the difference between approved medical charges and benefits paid by Medicare.
    SYN: Medicare supplemental policy

meditation
    Concentration or focusing of attention for relaxation and other therapeutic effects.

member
    Person covered by a health maintenance organization, including employee, spouse, children and other dependents.
    SYN: beneficiary
    SEE ALSO: enrollee
              insured
              subscriber

member month
A measure of HMO membership volume, defined as one member enrolled for one month in an HMO without regard to services received.

membership change
The amendment of the bylaws or articles of incorporation of a non-profit organization to reflect a modification in membership.

memorandum of understanding (MOU)
A written agreement outlining the tentative terms of a proposed transaction, pending matters still to be resolved or negotiated.

merger
A transaction in which one or more corporations are subsumed by another through the acquisition of assets and liabilities. One company becomes the survivor, while the merged company ceases to have an independent existence.
SEE ALSO: consolidation

MERP
medical expense reimbursement plan

MET
multiple employer trust

method
The orderly sequence of events of a process or procedure.

MEWA
multiple employer welfare association

MFM
maternal and fetal medicine

MFS
1. maxillofacial surgery
2. medical fee schedule

mg
milligram

MGMA
Medical Group Management Association

MH
mental health

MHCA
Managed Health Care Association

MH-SA
mental health-substance abuse

MHSS
military health services system

MI
1. medically indigent
2. myocardial infarction (heart attack)

MIB
medical information bureau

MIC
maternal and infant care

microscopic anatomy
The study of the structure of cells, tissue, and organs with the use of a light microscope.
SEE: histology

midwife
A person who assists with routine labor and delivery of newborns, and cares for the infant after birth.

midwife, nurse
SEE: nurse midwife

MIG
medicare-insured group

minimally invasive surgery
An operation performed with needles, catheters, or endoscopic instruments inserted through small incisions in the skin.
SYN: closed surgery
SEE ALSO: noninvasive
open surgery

MIP
managed indemnity plan

MIS
management information system

miscellaneous services
SEE: ancillary services

mix, contract
SEE: contract mix

mixed-model health maintenance organization
A health plan that includes more than one type of physician practice, for example a staff-model HMO that also contracts with independent physicians (IPAs) or group practices.

ml
milliliter

MLP
mid-level practitioner

MLR
medical loss ratio

mm
millimeter

MM
1. major medical
2. medical microbiology
3. member months

MOB
1. maintenance of benefits
2. medical office building

mobility
The ability of the patient to go outdoors, with mechanical assistance if needed.

model, actuarial cost
SEE: actuarial cost model

model, foundation
  SEE: foundation model

modified community rating
  SEE: community rating
      experience rating

modified duty
  SEE: modified work duty

modified fee-for-service
  A system of reimbursing physicians that combines fee-for-service with maximum payable limits for specific procedures or services.

modified work duty
  A program that involves making physical changes and alterations in the normal chores and responsibilities, that permits a disabled person to return to work while he or she recovers, although not in the identical capacity as before the illness or injury.
  SYN: modified duty
  SEE: return-to-work program
      work hardening

monitoring
  The continual, systematic collection and analysis of information about patient care, and its comparison against an established level of performance.

MOR
  monthly operating report

morbidity
  The occurrence of illness.

morbidity rate
  1. The number of cases of an injury, illness or condition within a given time period, usually a year.
  2. The ratio of sick persons to well persons in a defined population.

morgue technician
> *SEE:* diener

mortality
> The death of a patient.

mortality rate
> The proportion of deaths in a defined population of patients.

most-favored nation
> A provision in health care contracting requiring a provider to offer the other party to the contract the lowest price charged to any payer.

MOU
> memorandum of understanding

MP
> 1. medical payment
> 2. minimum premium

MPP
> minimum premium plan

MRA
> magnetic resonance angiography

MRI
> 1. magnetic resonance imaging
> 2. Medical Records Institute

MS
> 1. multiple sclerosis
> 2. musculoskeletal

MSA
> 1. medical savings account
> 2. metropolitan statistical area

MSH
> melanocyte-stimulating hormone

MSO
> 1. medical staff organization
> 2. management services organization

multidisciplinary
Calling upon the expertise of two or more specialized areas.

multiple births
Two or more newborns delivered without complications.

multiple choice
SEE: dual option

multiple employer trust (MET)
An organization authorized by federal law to provide benefits for two or more employer groups.

multiple employer welfare arrangement (MEWA)
A welfare plan to provide benefits for employees of two or more employers.

multispecialty group
A medical group practice of physicians in two or more clinical specialties.

music therapy
The use of music for therapeutic purposes.

MVP
mitral valve prolapse

MWEA
SEE: multiple employer welfare arrangement

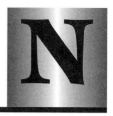

N
neurology

NAAC
National Association for Ambulatory Care

NAACLS
National Accrediting Agency for Clinical Laboratory Sciences

NACRH
National Advisory Committee on Rural Health

NAD
no acute distress

NAEBA
National Association of Employee Benefit Administrators

NAHC
National Association for Home Care

NAHQ
National Association for Healthcare Quality

NAIC
National Association of Insurance Commissioners

NAMCP
National Association of Managed Care Physicians

National Committee for Quality Assurance (NCQA)

national health insurance
A proposed unified government system to provide health insurance, similar to Medicare.

national health service
A proposed organization of providers employed by the federal government to render health and medical services.

natural death act
SEE: living will

naturopathic medicine
A philosophy of alternative medicine that emphasizes natural remedies.
SYN: naturopathy

naturopathy
SEE: naturopathic medicine

NB
newborn

NCHGR
National Center for Human Genome Research

NCI
1. National Cancer Institute
2. nursing care institution

NCPA
National Center for Policy Analysis

NCQA
National Committee for Quality Assurance

NCR
National Center for Research

NCRR
National Center for Research Resources

NCV
nerve conduction velocity

ND
neoplastic disease

NDC
National Drug Code

necessary treatment
    SEE: medically necessary

necessary, medically
    SEE: medically necessary

need, certificate of
    SEE: certificate of need

negligence
    The failure of a professional with a duty to act to provide the standard of care, which results in harm to a patient.
    SEE ALSO: duty to act
               malpractice
               standard of care

negligence, wanton
    SEE: wanton negligence

negligence, willful
    SEE: willful negligence

NEI
    National Eye Institute

neonatal period
    The first 28 days following birth, as used to calculate neonatal death rates and other statistics.

neonate, low birth weight
    SEE: low birth weight neonate

neonate, term
    SEE: term neonate

NEP
    nephrology

nephrologist
    A physician who specializes in diagnosing and treating kidney disorders.

nephrology
    The treatment of conditions and diseases affecting the kidneys.

net collection ratio
The proportion of a provider's net charges, after allowances and adjustments, that are collected in cash.

network
An affiliation of physicians, hospitals or other providers organized by an insurer or managed care company.

network, community care
SEE: community care network

network model HMO
A health maintenance organization that contracts with two or more independent group practices. Typically larger than a group model HMO.
SEE ALSO: health maintenance organization

network, primary care
SEE: primary care network

network provider
Physicians, hospitals, clinics, and other health professionals under contract to provide services to members of a managed care plan.
SYN: participating provider

network, provider services
SEE: provider services network

neurological surgery
The surgical treatment of conditions of the nervous system.
SYN: neurosurgery

neurologist
A physician who specializes in the diagnosis and nonsurgical treatment of conditions of the nervous system.

neurology
The nonsurgical treatment of conditions of the brain and nervous system.

neurosurgeon
A physician who specializes in the diagnosis and surgical treatment of diseases and injury of the brain and nervous system.

neurosurgery
SEE: neurological surgery

newborn admission
An infant who is hospitalized following birth.

newborn service day
The total health services received by a newborn patient in a 24-hour period.

newborn, well
SEE: well newborn

NG
nasogastric

NHB
National Health Board

NHLA
National Health Lawyers Association

NHLBI
National Heart, Lung and Blood Institute

NIA
National Institute on Aging

NIAAA
National Institute of Alcohol Abuse and Alcoholism

NIAID
National Institute of Allergy and Infectious Disease

NIAMSD
National Institute of Arthritis and Musculoskeletal and Skin Disorders

NICHHD
National Institute of Child Health and Human Development

NICU
neonatal intensive care unit

NIDA
National Institute on Drug Abuse

NIDCD
National Institute on Deafness and Other Communication Disorders

NIDDK
National Institute of Diabetes and Digestive and Kidney Diseases

NIDDM
non-insulin-dependent diabetes mellitus

NIDR
National Institute of Dental Research

NIEHS
National Institute of Environmental Health Sciences

NIGMS
National Institute of General Medical Sciences

NIH
National Institutes of Health

NIMH
National Institute of Mental Health

NINDS
National Institute of Neurological Disorders and Stroke

NINR
National Institute of Nursing Research

NIOSH
National Institute of Occupational Safety and Health

NKA
no known allergies

NKDA
no known drug allergies

NLM
National Library of Medicine

NLR
net loss ratio

NM
nuclear medicine

NMHA
National Mental Health Association

NMHCC
National Managed Health Care Congress

NMI
no middle initial

no-frills policy
SEE: bare-bones policy

no-shop clause
Provisions agreed to by parties of a proposed transaction that they will negotiate exclusively with each other and will not pursue another deal during a defined time period.
SYN: exclusive dealings clause

noc
night

nominal payment
SEE: token payment

non-accepting
A provider who does not participate in a given health care plan, such as Medicaid.
SYN: NON-PAR
SEE ALSO: non-participating provider

non-compliance
The failure of the patient to fulfill part or all of a treatment regimen prescribed by a physician or other health professional.
SEE ALSO: compliance

noncontributory
Not involved as a cause of a condition or result.

non-contributory plan
A health benefit plan in which the employer or sponsor pays 100% of the premium, without any contribution from the beneficiary.
SYN: medical expense reimbursement plan
SEE ALSO: contributory plan

non-core coverage
Health benefits other than standard core medical benefits, such as dental or vision care.
SEE ALSO: core coverage

non-disabling injury
Trauma that may require medical attention but does not cause time lost from work or serious impairment.

non-group insurance
SEE: individual insurance

noninvasive
Describing a diagnostic or therapeutic procedure that does not involve inserting an instrument or device through the skin or body orifice.
SEE ALSO: invasive

NON-PAR, nonpar
non-participating.
SEE: non-participating provider

nonparticipating provider
A provider without a contractual agreement with a health benefit plan to render care to eligible beneficiaries.
SYN: NON-PAR

nonprescription
SEE: over-the-counter

normal delivery
A newborn delivered without complications.

nosocomial disease
An illness or infection acquired in a hospital.
SYN: nosocomial infection

SEE ALSO: complication
iatrogenic disease

nosocomial infection
SEE: nosocomial disease

notice, admission
SEE: admission notification

NP
1. neuropathology
2. nurse practitioner

NPDB
National Practitioner Data Bank

NPH
neurophysiology

NPM
neonatal-perinatal medicine

NPO
nothing by mouth

NR
nuclear radiology

NRA
National Rehabilitation Association

NRHA
National Rural Health Association

NS
neurological surgery

NSR
normal sinus rhythm

nuclear medicine
The use of radioactive substances to diagnose and treat disease.

nuclear medicine physician
A medical doctor who specializes in the use of radioactive substances to diagnosis and treat disease.

nurse
An individual who has successfully completed the education, training, and testing requirements and is licensed by the state to practice nursing.

nurse anesthetist
A registered nurse with additional education and training who specializes in the administration of anesthesia during surgery.

nurse, circulating
SEE: circulating nurse

nurse clinician
SEE: nurse practitioner

nurse midwife
A nurse who has received additional training and assists with routine labor and delivery of normal newborns.

nurse practitioner
A registered nurse with advanced education and training who is responsible for providing primary or specialized health care services. Although nurse practitioners operate under the license of a medical doctor, they typically have a wide degree of autonomy and are often not directly supervised by a physician.

nurse, registered
SEE: registered nurse

nursing assistant
An individual who assists with patient care duties, such as feeding, bathing, and monitoring of vital signs, but does not administer medications.
SYN: nursing extender

nursing extender
SEE: nursing assistant

nursing home
A facility that provides skilled nursing care to elderly residents 24 hours a day.
SYN: domiciliary care
home for the aged

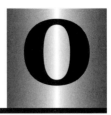

O
Objective

OAM
Office of Alternative Medicine

OB-GYN, OB/GYN
obstetrics and gynecology

OBG
obstetrics and gynecology

OBRA
Omnibus Budget Reconciliation Act

OBS
obstetrics

observation patient
A patient with signs and symptoms of a condition that may require hospitalization, who is held for monitoring and further assessment before a determination is made to either admit, discharge, or refer to another facility.

obstetrician
A physician who specializes in assisting with the delivery of newborns.

obstetrics
The care and treatment of the mother and child during pregnancy, childbirth and the immediate postpartum period.

obstetrics and gynecology (OB-GYN, OB/GYN)
The medical field related to the diagnosis and treatment of the female reproductive system, and care of the mother and fetus during pregnancy and childbirth.

occupational therapy
The rehabilitation of physically or emotionally disabled patients with tasks intended to improve function and the ability to cope with the demands of daily life.

occurrence screen
The review of medical records and patient care based on one or more events indicating a potential problem.

OCL
outstanding claims liability

OD
1. Doctor of Optometry
2. overdose
3. right eye

off-label prescribing
The practice of prescribing medication for indications that are not formally approved by the Food and Drug Administration, such as experimental treatments.
SYN: off-label use

off-label use
SEE: off-label prescribing

offset, behavior
SEE: behavior offset

OH
occupational history

OHMO
Office of Health Maintenance Organizations

OM
occupational medicine

OMAR
Office of Medical Applications Research

OMSB
Outcomes Management Standards Board

ONC
medical oncology

on call
SEE: call

oncologist
A physician who specializes in the diagnosis and treatment of cancer.

oncology
The science studying the cause, diagnosis and treatment of cancer.

one-day surgery
SEE: ambulatory surgery

OOA
out of area

OON
out of network

OOP
out of pocket

OP
outpatient

open access
SEE: open panel

open access HMO
SYN: open-ended HMO
SEE: point-of-service plan

open-ended HMO
SYN: open access HMO
SEE: hybrid managed care
point-of-service plan

open enrollment
A period of time in which insurers and health plans accept new applicants. Open enrollment periods are held once or twice annually to allow a change in health benefits.

open panel
A health benefit plan in which managed care companies contract with private physicians to provide services in their own offices. Usually, physicians are permitted to see other private, non-HMO patients as well.
SEE ALSO: closed panel

open staff
A network of providers that accepts new patients.

open surgery
An operative procedure in which internal structures of the body are exposed by incisions in the skin and superficial tissues.
SEE ALSO: minimally invasive surgery

operating margin
The difference between operating expenses and operating revenue, expressed as a percentage.

operating room (OR)
A hospital department with equipment and staff set up to perform surgical procedures.

operation
A surgical procedure.
SEE ALSO: surgery

OPH
ophthalmology

OPHC
Office of Prepaid Health Care

OPHCOO
Office of Prepaid Health Care Operations and Oversight

OPL
other party liability

OPM
Office of Personnel Management

opt-out
> An option available in some managed care plans that allows patients to seek care from a non-network provider, usually at a lower level of coverage, such as a point-of-service (POS) plan or a preferred provider organization (PPO).
> *SEE ALSO:* point-of-service plan

option, sole-source
> *SEE:* sole-source option

option, triple
> *SEE:* triple option

OR
> operating room

organ
> An organization of one or more tissues which collectively perform specific functions, such as respiration or digestion.
> *SEE ALSO:* system
> tissue

organization, health maintenance
> *SEE:* health maintenance organization

organization, management services
> *SEE:* management services organization

organization, peer review
> *SEE:* peer review organization

organization, pharmacy services administration
> *SEE:* pharmacy services administration organization

organization, physician-hospital community
> *SEE:* physician-hospital community organization

organization, professional review
> *SEE:* professional review organization

organization, professional standards review
> *SEE:* professional standards review organization

organization, utilization review
> *SEE:* utilization review organization

organ procurement
The process of obtaining organs or tissue for transplantation.

ORIF
open reduction, internal fixation

ORS
orthopaedic surgery

orthomolecular therapy
An alternative medicine that claims beneficial effects by altering the concentration of vitamins and other nutrients in the body, generally by encouraging large "megadoses."

ORWH
Office of Research for Women's Health

OS
left eye

OSC
organized system of care

OSCR
on-site concurrent review

OSHA
Occupational Safety and Health Administration

osteopathy
A philosophy that combines manipulative therapies with traditional medical management of disease, generally with a holistic approach.

OT
1. occupational therapist
2. occupational therapy
3. otology

OTC
over-the-counter

OTO
otolaryngology

OU
both eyes

out-of-area (OOA)
1. Outside of the service area of a managed care plan.
2. Provisions for health coverage when a member is outside a managed care plan's service area.

out-of-network referral
The direction of a patient to a provider or facility not within an approved panel. Care may be covered at a lower level than in-network services.

out-of-pocket cap
The maximum limit an insured patient must pay in the form of deductibles and copayments.

out-of-pocket costs (OOP)
Money paid by the patient for medical products and services, such as deductibles, copayments and coinsurance.

outcome
The consequences of medical care on an individual or group of patients.

outcome, clinical
SEE: clinical outcome

outcome, intermediate
SEE: intermediate outcome

outcome measure
An endpoint or factor used to evaluate medical care, such as survival, discharge status, or quality of life.

outcomes management
The improvement of patient care through the empirical study of treatment and the development of clinical protocols.
SEE ALSO: practice guidelines

outcomes research
Evaluation of specific health services in terms of costs and impact on the patient.

outlier

1. A patient whose course of treatment is significantly different than other similar patients, for example in terms of costs or in length of stay in the hospital.
2. Datum more than two standard deviations from the mean.

outlier, cost
> *SEE:* cost outlier

outlier, day
> *SEE:* stay outlier

outlier, stay
> *SEE:* stay outlier

outpatient care
Medical services that are provided without the need for an overnight stay in a hospital, such as through an ambulatory care clinic or emergency department.
> *SEE ALSO:* inpatient care

outpatient facility
> *SEE:* ambulatory care facility

outpatient facility, affiliated
> *SEE:* affiliated outpatient facility

outpatient, hospital
> *SEE:* hospital outpatient

outpatient surgery
> *SEE:* ambulatory surgery

outpatient surgery center
A facility for performing minor surgical procedures without the need for admitting the patient for an overnight stay in a hospital.
> *SEE ALSO:* ambulatory surgery

outpatient visit
> *SEE:* encounter

outside consultant
A medical specialist who is not a member of a managed care network

outside referral
The referral of a patient to a provider who is not on the staff of an HMO or within its network.

over-the-counter (OTC)
Medications and devices sold without a prescription.
SYN: nonprescription

overbilling
The practice of billing separately for unbundled procedures, services not performed, or failing to disclose patient copayments.

overcoding
The practice by providers of reporting a procedure that is more complex or expensive than actually performed.
SYN: code creep
SEE ALSO: gaming the system
upcoding

overhead, allocation of
SEE: allocation of overhead

overutilization
The delivery of health services at a frequency or level greater than medically necessary.

oxidative therapy
An alternative medicine claimed to produce a therapeutic effect by administering substances believed to increase the availability of oxygen in the body, such as with hydrogen peroxide or ozone therapy.

oz
ounce

ozone therapy
An alternative medicine which holds that a beneficial effect is produced by the administration of ozone.

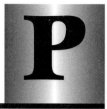

P
1. plan
2. posterior
3. psychiatry
4. pulse

P&A
protection and advocacy

PA
1. clinical pharmacology
2. physician's assistant
3. posterior anterior

package pricing
The establishment of a single bundled price for all medical and professional services related to a procedure or diagnosis.
SEE ALSO: global pricing

PAHO
Pan-American Health Organization

paid claims loss ratio (PCLR)
The liability for claims that are incurred and paid within a specified time period, divided by premiums received by a health plan.

pain and suffering cap
A limitation placed on the financial compensation that may be awarded for emotional distress suffered as the result of medical malpractice.

palliative
Providing relief from symptoms, but having no effect on underlying disease.

palliative care
Medical treatment to reduce the severity of symptoms without curing the underlying disease or condition.

palpated
Touched with the fingers and hands, usually for diagnostic purposes.

palpation
The use of the hands and fingers to feel objects beneath the surface of the skin.

pandemic
A disease affecting populations within an extensive geographic region.
> SEE ALSO: endemic
> epidemic

panel, closed
> SEE: closed panel

panel, open
> SEE: open panel

paneled
Referring to a provider who is contracted with a health maintenance organization.

Pap
Papanicolaou smear or test

PAR
postanesthetic recovery

paradigm
A model or mind-set for understanding.

paralysis
The loss of ability to move part or all of one's body.

paramedic
A prehospital care provider with more advanced training than an emergency medical technician. Paramedics typically are

permitted to intubate, administer medications and use other life-support measures.

SYN: advanced emergency medical technician
SEE ALSO: emergency medical technician
EMT-A

paraplegia
The loss of ability to move the lower extremities, often with a loss of sensation as well. Commonly caused by trauma or disease to the spinal cord.

paraprofessional
An individual who assists with the performance of a professional's duties.
SEE ALSO: allied health personnel

parenteral
Referring to the administration of a medication or other substance by a means other than the gastrointestinal tract, such as intramuscular or intravenous injection.

Part A, Medicare
SEE: Medicare Part A

Part B, Medicare
SEE: Medicare Part B

partial disability
The inability to perform some of one's usual work duties due to a medical condition.
SEE ALSO: total disability

partial hospitalization
An arrangement in which patients spend part of their time in the hospital, with the remainder in the community on day- or overnight passes. Employed while patients are transitioned to less-intensive supervision and care, such as during the recovery after hospitalization for mental illness or substance abuse.

participant
SEE: beneficiary

participating medical group (PMP)
> A medical group practice with a contractural arrangement with a managed care company or third-party payer.

participating provider
> 1. A provider who agrees to always accept Medicare's approved amount as the full charge for services rendered.
> 2. A provider who will bill a health insurance carrier directly, and bill the patient for the balance not paid by the insurer.
> *SYN:* network provider

participation
> A contractual arrangement by which a provider agrees to the compensation terms of a health benefit plan.

partnership
> Two or more people who co-own a business for profit.
> *SEE ALSO:* corporation
> sole proprietorship

PAS
> 1. professional activities survey
> 2. preadmission screening

PAT
> preadmission testing

pathologic histologist
> *SEE:* histopathologist

pathologic histology
> *SEE:* histopathology

pathway, clinical
> *SEE:* treatment protocol

pathway, critical
> *SEE:* critical pathway

patient
> 1. A person who suffers from an illness or injury.
> 2. A person who receives health care services.
> *SYN:* health care consumer
> *SEE ALSO:* inpatient
> outpatient

patient assessment
SEE: work-up

patient care manager
SEE: gatekeeper

patient compliance
SEE: compliance

patient day
SEE: inpatient services day

patient days
The number of patients hospitalized in a medical facility at a given time, such as midnight.
SEE ALSO: inpatient services day

patient dumping
The denial of medical care, such as by transfer or discharge, because of financial considerations rather than medical necessity.
SEE ALSO: anti-dumping law
Consolidated Omnibus Budget Reconciliation Act of 1985

patient, hospital
SEE: hospital patient

patient, limited-stay
SEE: short-stay patient

patient pathways
SEE: treatment protocol

patient protection law
SEE: any willing provider

patient record, electronic
SEE: electronic patient record

patient, observation
SEE: observation patient

patient, short-stay
SEE: short-stay patient

patients, ward
> *SEE*: ward patients

payer
> An organization, employer, insurer, government or individual who pays for health care or medical services.
> *SYN*: payor

payer mix
> The profile of a patient population based on the category of payor, including Medicare, Medicaid, Blue Cross-Blue Shield, commercial carrier, and self-pay.

payment, fixed
> *SEE*: fixed payment

payment, prospective
> *SEE*: prospective reimbursement

payment system, charge-based
> *SEE*: charge-based payment system

payment, token
> *SEE*: token payment

payor
> An outdated insurance industry term for the person or organization that ultimately pays for medical and health care services.
> *SYN*: payer

PC
> professional corporation

pc
> after meals

PCA
> 1. percutaneous angioplasty
> 2. patient-controlled analgesia

PCLR
> paid claims loss ratio

PCM
> pediatric critical care medicine

PCN
primary care network

PCP
1. primary care physician
2. primary care provider
3. phencyclidine (angel dust)

PCPM
per contract per month

PCR
1. physician contingency reserve
2. polymerase chain reaction

PD
pediatrics

PDA
1. pediatric allergy
2. patent ductus arteriosus

PDC
pediatric cardiology

PDE
pediatric endocrinology

PDP
1. pediatric pulmonology
2. pediatric pathology

PDR
1. Physician's Desk Reference
2. pediatric radiology

PDS
pediatric surgery

PE
physical examination

PEC
pre-existing condition

peds
pediatrics

peer grouping
The classification of health care facilities into groups with similar characteristics, such as number of beds, patient mix, location, medical school affiliation, or profit/nonprofit status.

peer review
1. The process through which physicians evaluate the quality of health care services provided by a managed care organization.
2. The critique of reports and papers by experts prior to publication in professional journals.

peer review organization (PRO)
Groups of health professionals contracted by Medicare to evaluate the necessity and quality of health services provided to Medicare beneficiaries.

PEFR
peak expiratory flow rate

PEM
pediatric emergency medicine

per
by

per case rate
SEE: case rate

per certification
Confirmation of a patient's eligibility for health benefits coverage by a third-party payer.

per contract per month (PCPM)

per diem
A daily rate paid to a medical facility for inpatient medical care. May be bundled with physician fees and other professional services in managed care contracts.
SYN: daily rate

perfect stay
A hospitalization without unnecessary care.

performance measure
The evaluation of how well a health care system serves a population of beneficiaries, such as rates of mammography or colorectal cancer screening, frequency of physical exams, or patient satisfaction.

performance standards, volume
SEE: volume performance standards

per member per month (PMPM)
A method of calculating premiums or capitation rates by health plans, particularly health maintenance organizations (HMOs). The per member per month rate is the amount of money contractually agreed upon in a prepaid health plan.

period, benefit
SEE: benefit period

period, elimination
SEE: elimination period

period, experience
SEE: experience period

period, neonatal
SEE: neonatal period

permanent disability
The limitation or impairment of a person's ability to perform the ordinary duties of work for a period in excess of one year, and may persist for the remainder of the individual's life.

PERRLA
Pupils equal, round, and reactive to light and accommodation.

person, affected
SEE: affected person

person, covered
SEE: covered person

personal identification
A unique number assigned to patients for the purposes of maintaining a medical record.

personal insurance
>   *SEE*: individual insurance

personnel, paramedical
>   *SEE*:· allied health personnel

per thousand members per year (PTMPY)
An indicator employed to measure hospital utilization.

PET
positron emission tomography

PF
peak flow

PFT
pulmonary function testing

PGE
pediatric gastroenterology

PGP
prepaid group practice

PH
1. past history
2. public health

Ph.D.
Doctor of philosophy

pharmaceutical care
Activities that enhance patient compliance with medication therapy, as a part of disease state management.
>   *SYN*: pharmacist care
>   *SEE*: disease state management

pharmacist care
>   *SEE*: pharmaceutical care

pharmacy services administration organization (PSAO)

phase I clinical trial
An experiment to test the safety of a new drug, procedure or process in human volunteer subjects.

phase II clinical trial
The evaluation of the effectiveness of a new drug or procedure in treating the condition for which it is intended.

phase III clinical trial
A comparison of a new drug or procedure against current treatment in human volunteer subjects.

PHCO
Physician-hospital community organization

PHO
1. pediatric hematology-oncology
2. physician-hospital organization

PHS
public health service

physiatrist
A physician who specializes in physical medicine and rehabilitation.

physiatry
The practice of physical medicine.

physical diagnosis
The determination of the nature of an illness by physical examination of the patient.

physical examination
The hands-on evaluation of a patient, including visual inspection, listening (auscultation), feeling (palpation), and percussion.

physical therapy
The treatment of musculoskeletal disorders, such as after injury or stroke, with physical conditioning, agents, exercise and methods.

physician
1. Person who is trained, qualified and licensed to practice medicine.
2. A doctor who practices medicine, as opposed to a surgeon.
   SYN: doctor
   medical doctor

physician assistant (PA)
Professional who provides health care under the supervision and guidance of a physician. Among the duties physician assistants perform are physical examinations, diagnostic testing, and the administration of medications, depending on applicable local and state laws.
SYN: physician extender

physician, attending
SEE: attending physician

physician contingency reserve (PCR)
SEE: withhold

physician extenders
All non-physician medical staff who care for patients in any setting, but particularly in hospitals, clinics and practice offices. Includes physician assistants (PAs) and other allied health professionals.
SEE ALSO: allied health personnel
physician assistant

physician-hospital community organization (PHCO)

physician-hospital organization (PHO)
A corporate entity jointly capitalized and owned by physicians and hospitals. Formed to negotiate managed care contracts with insurers and other third-party payers.

physician identification
A unique number assigned to physicians within a health care organization for medical records and information management systems.

physician, nuclear medicine
SEE: nuclear medicine physician

physician, primary care
SEE: primary care physician

physician profiling
SEE: credentialing

physiology
>The study of the processes and functions of the body and the response to disease or injury.

PI
>1. present illness
>2. principal investigator

PICU
>pediatric intensive care unit

PID
>1. pediatric infectious disease
>2. pelvic inflammatory disease

PIH
>pregnancy-induced hypertension

pink ladies
>*SEE*: volunteer

placebo
>1. An inert substance given as medicine for its suggestive effect.
>2. Inert material that is identical in appearance to a drug being tested in an experiment, in order to distinguish the drug effect from suggestion.
>*SYN*: sugar pill

placebo effect
>The subjective sense of improvement produced by suggestion following the administration of an inert substance or procedure which the recipient believes to be therapeutic.

plan, care
>*SEE*: care plan

plan, community care
>*SEE*: community care plan

plan, contract fee schedule
>*SEE*: contract fee schedule plan

plan, contributory
>*SEE*: contributory plan

plan, indemnity
> *SEE*: indemnity plan

plan, treatment
> *SEE*: treatment plan

play or pay
> A proposal mandating that employers give health insurance coverage to employees or pay a tax to finance a government-managed program to provide coverage to the uninsured.

PLI
> professional liability insurance

PM
> pain management

pm
> afternoon

PMA
> 1. pre-market approval
> 2. Pharmaceutical Manufacturers Association

PMH
> past medical history

PMP
> participating medical group

PMPM
> per member per month

PMPY
> per member per year

PMR
> physical medicine and rehabilitation

PNP
> pediatric nephrology

PNS
> peripheral nervous system

po
  by mouth

podiatric medicine
  SEE: podiatry

podiatrist
  A practitioner of podiatry.
  SYN: chiropodist
    podologist

podiatry
  The specialty concerned with the diagnosis and treatment of diseases, injuries and defects of the foot.
  SYN: chiropody
    podiatric medicine
    podology

podologist
  SEE: podiatrist

podology
  SEE: podiatry

point-of-service plan (POS)
  A benefit design with financial incentives to encourage patients to choose in-network providers, but which also allows for out-of-network health care services. For example, the patient may be required to pay a nominal copayment for care given by in-network providers, while coverage for non-network care is significantly reduced, subject to traditional deductibles and copayments.
  SYN: open-ended HMO
  SEE ALSO: health maintenance organization
    preferred provider organization
    hybrid managed care

points, trim
  SEE: trim points

policyholder
An individual covered by an insurance policy.
SYN: beneficiary
insured

policy, limited
SEE: limited policy

policy, rated
SEE: rated policy

pool, withhold
SEE: withhold pool

POP
premium-only plan

population
A group of people with common characteristics, traits or features.

population at risk
A group of people with one or more common characteristics that increase the chance of illness or injury.

population-based care
An approach to medicine involving the identification and treatment of conditions that affect specific groups of people.

portability
The guarantee of health benefit coverage without a waiting period or additional deductibles when an individual changes employers.

portable benefits
The ability to change employment without losing health care coverage, being subjected to a waiting period, or being excluded because of pre-existing conditions.
SYN: portability
SEE ALSO: job lock

POS
point of service

positron emission tomography (PET)

postop, post-op, post op
postoperative

postoperative (postop, post-op, post op)
After surgery.

postpartum
Referring to the period of time after birth.

post-term infant
A neonate having 42 or more weeks of gestation.

power of attorney
A legal document which authorizes one person to make decisions on behalf of another. Does not apply to health care decisions.
SEE ALSO: durable power of attorney
health care proxy

PPBS
postprandial blood sugar

PPI-H
producer price index-hospital

PPO
preferred provider organization

PPO, first-generation
SEE: first-generation PPO

PPO, second-generation
SEE: second-generation PPO

PPO, third-generation
SEE: third-generation PPO

PPRC
Physician Payment Review Commission

PPS
prospective payment system

PR
by rectum

practice, contract
    SEE: contract practice

practice, family
    SEE: family practice

practice, group
    SEE: group practice

practice guideline
    SEE: treatment protocol

practice guidelines
    Written recommendations for the most appropriate diagnostic procedures and treatments for specified conditions.
    SYN: clinical pathway
           critical pathway
           protocol

practice parameter
    SEE: treatment protocol

practice parameters
    SEE: treatment protocol

practice plan, medical
    SEE: treatment protocol

practice policies
    SEE: treatment protocol

practice, solo
    SEE: solo practice

practice standards
    SEE: treatment protocol

pranic healing
    A form of alternative medicine involving the assessment of an "aura," or energy field, believed to surround the body.

preadmission certification
    The evaluation of a request for admission to a hospital and the determination of medical necessity based on established criteria.

SYN: preadmission review
SEE ALSO: prospective review
     utilization management

preadmission review
SEE: preadmission certification

preadmission testing (PAT)
Radiologic and laboratory tests that are performed before a patient is admitted to the hospital.

preauthorization
Approval granted by the primary care provider or managed care company prior to treatment. A means of managing the utilization of care.
SYN: pre-cert
SEE ALSO: gatekeeper
     predetermination
     prospective review
     utilization management

precautions, universal
SEE: universal precautions

pre-cert
SEE: preauthorization

precipitate delivery
SEE: emergency childbirth

predetermination
A provision of some benefit plans requiring providers to submit a treatment plan to the third-party payer for administrative review. Typically used when covered charges are expected to exceed a specified amount.
SEE ALSO: prospective review

preemie
An infant born before the normal length of gestation.
SYN: premature infant
SEE ALSO: preterm infant

preemption

pre-established criteria
Written, accepted standards of care.

pre-existing condition (PEC)
An illness or injury acquired by the patient prior to enrollment in a health benefit plan. Technically, any illness for which a newly insured person has been treated during a period of time, such as the previous 6–12 months. Pre-existing conditions may be excluded from coverage temporarily or permanently, or may disqualify an applicant from membership.

preferred provider
A hospital, physician or other licensed health professional with a contractual arrangement with a managed care health benefit plan.

preferred provider organization (PPO)
An arrangement in which a network of physicians, hospitals and other providers agree to render care on a fee-for-service basis, using a fee schedule or a discount from usual and customary rates. May also employ credentialing, utilization management and other managed care strategies. Patients are encouraged to see providers within the network with financial incentives such as lower out-of-pocket costs.

premature infant
SEE: preemie
preterm infant

premium
A periodic payment entitling a person to health care services covered by insurance or benefit plan.

premium, contributory
SEE: contributory premium

premium-only plan (POP)

premium, waiver of
SEE: waiver of premium

premium, written
    SEE: written premiums

prenatal diagnosis
    The detection of diseases and malformation prior to birth.

pre op
    preoperative

preop, pre-op
    preoperative

preoperative (preop, pre-op)
    Before surgery.

prepaid group practice
    A group of physicians or other providers under contract to an HMO or other managed care plan to provide health care services to a group of subscribers.
    SEE ALSO: health maintenance organization
        prospective payment

prepaid health care
    An arrangement in which managed care companies pay providers prior to the delivery of health care services, such as in a health maintenance organization. Typically, the payment is capitated, e.g., a flat rate per member per month.
    SYN: prepayment
        prospective payment

prepayment
    SEE: prospective reimbursement

prescribing, off-label
    SEE: off-label prescribing

preterm infant
    A neonate weighing 1,000 to 2,499 grams at birth and/or having a gestation of 28 to 37 weeks.
    SYN: preemie
        premature infant

prevailing fee
The fee level most often charged for health care services in a given area.
SEE ALSO: reasonable fee
SYN: customary fee
   fee screen
   prevailings
   usual fee

prevailings
SEE: prevailing fee

prevalence
The number of cases of a disease within a population within a defined time period.
SEE ALSO: incidence

prevention, tertiary
SEE: tertiary prevention

preventive medicine
Health care activities intended to protect against the development of disease or disability. Involves services to avoid disease (e.g., immunization), screening to detect disease early (e.g., Pap smears, mammography), and interventions to prevent deterioration of the patient's condition (e.g., physical therapy).
SYN: preventive services
SEE ALSO: community medicine
   health education
   public health

preventive services
SEE: preventive medicine

price, average wholesale
SEE: average wholesale price

pricing, package
SEE: package pricing

pricing, shadow
SEE: shadow pricing

primal scream therapy
> *SEE*: primal therapy

primal therapy
> A form of psychotherapy involving the identification and resolution of repressed pain and emotions.
> *SYN*: primal scream therapy

primary care
> Basic, general health care services that are intended to prevent disease, detect illness at an early stage, and to treat routine, uncomplicated conditions. Primary care is usually the patient's initial contact point with the health care system.
> *SEE ALSO*: secondary care
> tertiary care

primary care network (PCN)
> A group of primary care physicians organized into a formal entity with a contractual arrangement with a managed care company to provide services for members of a health benefit plan.

primary care physician (PCP)
> A physician who concentrates on family practice, internal medicine, general practice, pediatrics, or sometimes obstetrics and gynecology (OB/GYN), who acts as the primary manager of patient care for an enrollee in a health maintenance organization (HMO) or preferred provider organization (PPO).
> *SYN*: gatekeeper
> *SEE ALSO*: managed care
> primary care provider

primary care provider
> *SEE*: gatekeeper
> primary care physician

principal diagnosis
> The condition responsible for a hospitalization, determined by evaluation of the patient.

principal procedure
A procedure primarily performed to treat the patient's condition, rather than to assist in diagnosis or other reasons.

Pritikin diet
A dietary regimen that emphasizes unrefined, fiber-rich foods and eschews fats and highly refined carbohydrates. Often used with aerobic exercise.

privilege, attorney-client
SEE: attorney-client privilege

privileging, clinical
SEE: clinical privileging

privileges
SEE: clinical privileges

prn
as needed

PRO
peer review organization

pro bono
SEE: charity care

procedure
A specific action, process or test performed for the diagnosis or treatment of a patient.

procedure, auxiliary
SEE: auxiliary procedure

procedure code
SEE: current procedural terminology

procedure, incidental
SEE: incidental procedure

procedure, invasive
SEE: invasive

procedure, noninvasive
SEE: noninvasive

procedure, principal
> *SEE*: principal procedure

procedures, grievance
> *SEE*: grievance procedures

procedure, significant
> *SEE*: significant procedure

process management team
> A group of professionals in a quality improvement program.

proctology
> The treatment of conditions of the colon and rectum.
> *SYN*: colon and rectal surgery

prodromal period
> *SEE*: incubation period

producer price index-hospital (PPI-H)

professional courtesy
> Free or discounted services provided by physicians or other health professionals to their colleagues.

professional liability insurance (PLI)
> *SYN*: malpractice insurance

professional staff
> Attending physicians affiliated with a hospital.

professional standards review organization (PSRO)

prognosis
> A prediction of the likely outcome of a disease based on the health status of the patient and knowledge of the typical course of the illness or condition.

program, employee assistance
> *SEE*: employee assistance program

program, incentive
> *SEE*: incentive program

program, rehabilitation
> *SEE*: rehabilitative services

program, return-to-work
SEE: return-to-work program

project home
SEE: assisted living facility

ProPAC
Prospective Payment Assessment Commission

prophylaxis
A process or intervention taken to prevent disease or some other consequence.

prospective
Before the fact; looking forward.
SEE: retrospective

prospective payment
SEE: prepaid health care
prospective reimbursement

prospective reimbursement
A method of compensating hospitals, physicians and other health care providers before services are provided. Typically a capitated rate of payment that is determined in advance.
SYN: prepaid health care
SEE ALSO: at-risk contracting
capitation
prepaid health care
prepayment
prospective payment

prospective review
An evaluation of health care services to be performed before they are delivered, often involving pre-admission certification before admission to a hospital, or preauthorization of surgery.
SEE ALSO: concurrent review
retrospective review

prosthesis
An artificial substitute for a diseased or missing limb or body part.

prosthetics
The art and science of making and maintaining artificial human body parts, such as limbs.
SEE ALSO: orthotics

protection and advocacy (P&A)

protocol, treatment
SEE: treatment protocol

provider
A physician, nurse, hospital, clinic, or other health professional or facility.

provider, contract
SEE: contract provider

provider, network
SEE: network provider

provider, nonparticipating
SEE: nonparticipating provider

provider, participating
SEE: participating provider

provider, preferred
SEE: preferred provider

provider, primary care
SEE: primary care physician

provider services network
A proposed type of provider-sponsored prepaid health plan, similar to a health maintenance organization (HMO) but it is not required to fulfill all of the regulatory capital and reserve requirements in force for licensed HMO plans in each state.

provisional diagnosis
SEE: admission diagnosis

provision, comparability
SEE: comparability provision

provision, reinstatement
>   *SEE*: reinstatement provision

PS
>   plastic surgery

PSA
>   prostate-specific antigen

PSAO
>   Pharmacy Services Administration Organization

PSG
>   polysomnography

PSN
>   provider services network

PSRO
>   Professional Standards Review Organization

psychiatrist
>   A medical doctor who specializes in the diagnosis and treatment of mental illness.

psychiatrist, child
>   *SEE*: child psychiatrist

psychiatry
>   The medical specialty concerned with the diagnosis and treatment of mental illness.

psychic surgery
>   A form of health fraud in which practitioners claim to perform surgery by unconventional means, such as with the bare hands.

psychologist
>   A health professional, usually with a Ph.D., licensed to practice psychology.

psychology
>   The profession and practice concerned with human behavior and related mental processes.

psychosocial services
Mental health care addressing the psychological and social needs of patients.

psychotherapy
The treatment of emotional, behavioral, personality or psychiatric disorders primarily through verbal and non-verbal communication with the patient, rather than with medication or physical interventions.

pt
patient

PT
1. physical therapy
2. physical therapist
3. prothrombin time

PTCA
percutaneous transluminal coronary angioplasty

PTH
1. parathyroid hormone
2. anatomic/clinical pathology

PTMPY
per thousand members per year

PTT
partial thromboplastin time

public health
The scientific field concerned with the health status of communities, regions or nations. Public health issues include sanitation, control of infectious disease, vaccinations, population control, disease prevention, and injury control.

PUD
pulmonary diseases

puncture, lumbar
SEE: lumbar puncture

purchase discount
> SEE: contractual allowances

purchaser
> The sponsor of a health benefit plan, usually an employer, union or other group. The purchaser controls premium dollars and contracts with a health benefit organization to coverage for an enrolled population.

PV
> by vagina

Px
> physical examination

PYA
> psychoanalysis

PYM
> psychosomatic medicine

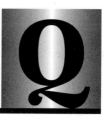

q
 every

QA
 quality assurance

qd
 every day

qh
 every hour

qid
 four times a day

qns
 quantity not sufficient

qod
 every other day

QIP
 quality improvement program

QMB
 Qualified Medicare beneficiary

QRC
 quality review committee

qs
 quantity sufficient

q2d
 every two hours

qualification, federal
 SEE: federal qualification

qualified administrator
A person who is currently licensed by the state in which he or she works, who is qualified to manage a long-term care facility.

qualified beneficiary
An individual covered by a health benefit plan who is eligible to receive health care services.

qualified child psychiatrist
SEE: child psychiatrist

qualified Medicare beneficiary (QMB)

quality
The degree to which health care services result in a desired patient outcomes.

quality assessment
The measurement of the quality of patient care at a given time.
SEE ALSO: quality assurance

quality assurance (QA)
The measurement of the level of patient care, and strategies to enhance quality when necessary.
SEE ALSO: quality assessment

quality improvement program (QIP)

quality review committee (QRC)

quality, total
SEE: total quality

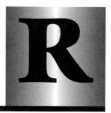

R
1. radiology
2. respiration
3. right

RAD
radiological physics

radiation therapy
SEE: x-ray therapy

RAF
risk adjustment factor

RAP
radiologists, anesthesiologists and pathologists

rate, attrition
SEE: attrition rate

rate, birth
SEE: birth rate

rate, composite
SEE: composite rate

rated policy
An insurance policy with a premium rate that is higher than standard due to additional risk, such as a health problem.
SYN: extra risk policy

rate, utilization
SEE: utilization rate

rating, experience
SEE: experience rating

rating, prospective
> *SEE:* prospective rating

ratio, acid test
> *SEE:* acid test ratio

ratio, cost-benefit
> *SEE:* cost-benefit ratio

ratio, medical loss
> *SEE:* medical loss ratio

RBC
> 1. red blood cell
> 2. red blood count

RBRVS
> resource-based relative value scale

R&C
> reasonable and customary charges

RCE
> reasonable compensation equivalent

RCF
> residential care facility

RD
> registered dietitian

reaction
> 1. The action of antibody on antigen.
> 2. The interaction of two or more chemicals, forming new substances.
> 3. The response of living tissue or an organism to a stimulus.

readmission
> The admission of a patient to an inpatient medical facility shortly after discharge, often to care for conditions related to the original admission.

readmission rate
> The proportion of patients who are rehospitalized among a defined population, such as those with a specific diagnosis or members of a particular health plan.

reagent
> A substance added to a solution to produce a chemical reaction.

recap sheet, daily
> *SEE:* daily recap sheet

record, variation
> *SEE:* variation record

recovery, service
> *SEE:* service recovery

recurrent
> Referring to symptoms or conditions that reappear after a period of absence.
> *SEE ALSO:* remission

recurring clause
> Provisions defining the time period within which the recurrence of a condition is considered a continuation of a previous episode of health care use, rather than a new episode.

redlining
> The practice of denying insurance coverage to applicants within a defined geographic area.
> *SEE ALSO:* industrial screening
> blacklisting

red rules
> Strict policies or regulations that cannot be violated.
> *SEE ALSO:* blue rules

reference
> *SEE:* benchmark

referenced diagnostic services
> The performance of hospital laboratory or other diagnostic testing for patients cared by physicians in the community and not admitted to the hospital.

referral
The process by which a patient is directed by a primary care physician for evaluation and treatment by a specialist or clinical facility.

referral, out-of-network
SEE: out-of-network referral

referral, outside
SEE: outside referral

referral provider
SEE: referral specialist

referral specialist
A specialist who cares for patients referred by a primary care provider.
SYN: referral provider
SEE ALSO: specialist, referral

reflex
An involuntary reaction to stimulation of the peripheral nerves. Tested as part of a neurological assessment.

reflexology
A form of massage therapy based on the belief that specific points on the palms of the hands or soles of the feet correspond to internal organs.
SYN: zone therapy

refund, experience
SEE: experience refund

regional alliance
SEE: alliance

registered nurse (RN)

rehab
SEE: rehabilitation

rehabilitation
The physical and emotional restoration of a patient following illness or injury.
SYN: rehab

rehabilitation, cardiac
SEE: cardiac rehabilitation

rehabilitation program
A comprehensive, coordinated service that assists patients to reach the maximal level of recovery following severe injury or illness. Typically includes physical medicine, social services, and vocational services.

rehabilitation, vocational
SEE: vocational rehabilitation

Reichian therapy
A type of massage therapy intended to break down emotional "armor" and enhance sexual energy.

reimbursement, cost
See: cost reimbursement

reimbursement, cost-based
SEE: cost-based reimbursement

reimbursement, direct
SEE: direct reimbursement

reimbursement, prospective
SEE: prospective reimbursement

reimbursement, retrospective
SEE: cost-based reimbursement

reimbursement, third-party
SEE: third-party reimbursement

reinstatement
The resumption of coverage under a health benefit policy that had lapsed or been revoked.

reinstatement provision
Terms under which a health benefit plan may be reissued after a policy has lapsed.

reinsurance
Insurance policies obtained by self-insured employers, HMOs and other health benefit plans to cover potential costs, such as out-of-area services. Often used to pay large claims for an individual or in aggregate for an employer group.
> *SYN:* excess-of-loss insurance
> *SEE ALSO:* stop-loss
> stop-loss insurance

release of information
A document recording the patient's informed consent for medical information to be disclosed to an employer, insurer, managed care company, attorney or other third party.
> *SEE ALSO:* patient confidentiality
> informed consent

reliability
The reproducibility of findings, yielding similar results with repeated testing.
> *SEE ALSO:* validity

remission
A period during the course of a disease when symptoms are lessened or abated, or when evidence of the disease is not present.

REN
reproductive endocrinology

replacement, single carrier
> *SEE ALSO:* single carrier replacement

report, variance
> *SEE:* variance report

request for information (RFI)

request for proposal (RFP)

required services
> *SEE:* mandated services

research, basic
 SEE: basic research

research, clinical
 SEE: clinical research

research, outcomes
 SEE: outcomes research

reserve, physician contingency
 SEE: physician contingency reserve

resident
 1. A person who lives within a defined geographic area.
 2. A person who lives in a facility, such as a group home.
 3. A physician who has completed medical school and is performing one or more years of training in a specialty area.
 SYN: house staff

resident day
 SEE: resident services day

resident services day
 The sum of all health care services provided to a resident in a health care facility in one 24-hour period.
 SYN: resident day

residential care facility (RCF)
 A housing arrangement to provide custodial care for persons who are unable to live independently because of emotional, mental or physical disabilities.
 SYN: group home
 SEE ALSO: custodial care
  rest home
  skilled nursing facility

residual market
 High-risk small employers who are unable to obtain workers' compensation health insurance coverage. Typically covered by a shared risk pool or a state system.
 SEE ALSO: shared risk pool

respite care
Health services intended to provide relief for family care-givers of patients with long-term illness. Respite care is usually on a short-term basis, from a few hours to several days.

rest home
An inpatient residential facility that provides custodial care only. While some rest homes may offer limited nursing services, the level of care is generally less intense than provided in an intermediate care facility.
SEE ALSO: intermediate care facility

restrictions
SEE: limitations

retention
1. The portion of a cost of a health benefit plan that is allocated by the insurer or managed care company to cover administrative costs and profit.
2. The portion of expected losses or payments that an employer chooses to self-fund rather than to insure.
SEE ALSO: administrative load

retrospective
After the fact; looking backward.
SEE ALSO: prospective

retrospective analysis
A review of data related to events or transactions in the past.
SEE ALSO: concurrent review
prospective review
retrospective review

retrospective reimbursement
The payment of providers after care has been rendered to patients, based on actual charges, a schedule of fees, or some other arrangement.
SEE ALSO: cost-based reimbursement
prospective payment

retrospective review
An evaluation of care performed and charges billed after services have been rendered, based on the collection and analysis of data from the patient record.
SEE ALSO: prospective review

return-to-work program
A program designed to assist an injured or ill employee resume a regular or modified job while recovery continues.

review board, institutional
SEE: institutional review board

review, claim
SEE: claim review

review, concurrent
SEE: concurrent review

review, continued stay
SEE: continued stay review

review, focused
SEE: focused review

review, peer
SEE: peer review

review, preadmission
SEE: preadmission certification

review, prospective
SEE: prospective review

review, retrospective
SEE: retrospective review

review, utilization
SEE: utilization review

RFI
request for information

RFP
request for proposal

RHCF
residential health care facility

RHI
rhinology

RHU
rheumatology

RIA
radioimmunoassay

rider
A provision added to an insurance policy that modifies or extends coverage or benefits, such as the amount of coverage, exclusion of specific conditions, or the addition of mental health coverage.

rider, cost of living
SEE: cost of living rider

right-to-die
A philosophy that competent persons with terminal illness have a right to refuse health care and other measures that postpone death.
SEE ALSO: living will

RIMS
Risk and Insurance Management Society

risk
The possibility of experiencing a financial loss.

risk-adjusted capitation
A method of compensating providers with a capitated rate that is modified to account for the health status of the group of patients being served.

risk adjustment
An additional amount paid in premiums when a group of members has a greater propensity for illness and more costly health care.
SYN: risk load

risk-bearing
Assuming responsibility for potential financial loss.

risk control
SEE: stop-loss

risk factor
A trait or characteristic that increases an individual's chance of experiencing diseases or injuries. Some risk factors, including smoking or a sedentary lifestyle, can be controlled. Other risk factors cannot, such as heredity, gender or age.
SEE ALSO: risk reduction

risk load
SEE: risk adjustment

risk measure
An estimation of the per capita costs of providing health care services to a group of individuals over a defined period of time.

risk pool
1. An amount of money set aside from provider compensation to cover health care expenses above certain targeted levels in a managed care plan. The pool is distributed if expenses are below specified levels, placing providers at risk.
SEE: at-risk contracting
2. A state-level program to provide health benefits to groups that are otherwise unable to obtain insurance in the commercial marketplace, such as high-risk occupations and small employers. The risks are usually shared among insurers who do business in the state.

risk shifting
A method by which providers share a portion of the liability for health care use and expenditures.

RLQ
right lower quadrant

RN
registered nurse

RO
radiation oncology

roadmap, clinical
SEE: clinical roadmap

Roentgen ray
SEE: x-ray

rolfing
An alternative form of massage and manipulation that links posture with well-being.
SYN: structural integration

R/O
rule out

ROM
Range of motion

room and board
The provision of a bed, meals, housekeeping, and other non-health services related to hospitalization.

room, operating
SEE: operating room

ROS
review of symptoms

rounds, ward
SEE: teaching rounds

roundtable
A health care coalition comprised of business and industry.

RP
1. radioisotopic pathology
2. retinitis pigmentosa
3. retrograde pyelogram

RRR
regular rate and rhythm

RTC
　return to clinic

RTO
　return to office

RTS
　repetitive trauma syndrome

rule, birthday
　　SEE: birthday rule

rule out (RO)
　Diagnostic procedures and treatments intended to eliminate possible causes of signs and symptoms, to arrive at a precise diagnosis.
　SEE ALSO: differential diagnosis

rules, blue
　　SEE: blue rules

rules, red
　　SEE: red rules

RUQ
　right upper quadrant

RVS
　1. relative value scale
　2. relative value of service

Rx
　recipe; prescription

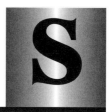

S
1. subjective
2. surgery

SA
1. sinoatrial
2. substance abuse

SAE
supplemental accident expense

safe harbors
Specific health care system configurations, relationships and activities that are permitted under federal antitrust laws.

SAMHSA
Substance and Mental Health Services Administration

sanitation, base
 SEE: base sanitation

SAP
service assessment program

satellite clinic
An outpatient care facility operated by a hospital that is located at a worksite or residential neighborhood to provide access to primary care and emergency services.

saturation
The maximum penetration of a health maintenance organization in a group or market.
 SEE ALSO: market share
     penetration

SB
    senate bill

SC
    services corporation

scale, sliding fee
    SEE: sliding fee scale

SCC
    surgical critical care

SCCM
    Society for Critical Care Medicine

schedule, benefit payment
    SEE: benefit payment schedule

schedule, call
    SEE: call schedule

schedule, fee
    SEE: fee schedule

schedule, indemnification
    SEE: table of allowances

schedule, surgical
    SEE: surgical schedule

Schuessler cell salts
    A group of homeopathic remedies believed to restore or enhance
    normal cellular physiology.
    SYN: tissue salts

SCR
    standard class rate

screen
    Criteria employed to select medical records for review.

screen, generic
    SEE: generic screen

screening
The administration of an inexpensive diagnostic test to large groups of predominantly asymptomatic individuals to identify those with a high risk of a given disease. Screening tests generally do not provide a specific diagnosis.

screening, health
SEE: health screening

screening, industrial
SEE: industrial screening

screen, occurrence
SEE: occurrence screen

SDU
step-down unit

secondary care
Medical interventions intended to prevent a worsening of condition or the development of complications in a patient suffering from illness or injury. Secondary care is often rendered by a specialist after referral from a primary care provider, and is usually less intensive than tertiary care.
SYN specialty care
SEE ALSO: primary care
tertiary care

second surgical opinion (SSO)

second-generation PPO
A PPO that includes case review, per-diem payment for hospitals, and physician reimbursement based on a relative-value fee schedule.
SEE ALSO: first-generation PPO
third-generation PPO

selection, adverse
SEE: adverse selection

self-care
The attendance to health care needs by the patient without the assistance of others.
SYN: self-help

self-funding
> *SEE:* self-insurance

self-help
> *SEE:* self-care

self-insurance
> An arrangement in which an employer or group assumes risk and pays for health care expenses usually covered by insurance.
> *SYN:* self-funding

self-referral
> 1. An option available in some health maintenance organizations to allow members to choose specialty care without referral by a primary care physician.
> 2. The selection of specialty care without formal approval by a managed care plan.

seniors' apartment
> An adults-only housing development typically offering services such as housekeeping, meals and organized activities.
> *SYN:* adults-only housing

sentinel event
> An adverse condition that could have been prevented by appropriate medical care, such as a hypertensive crisis that could have been avoided by proper medication and follow-up.

sequela
> A disorder or condition following, and usually resulting from a previous disease or injury.

service
> 1. Activities performed on behalf of others.
> 2. A unit of health care.
> *SEE ALSO:* clinical service
> health care service
> professional service

service area
> A defined geographic region in which an insurer or managed care company provides health care services for its enrollees.
> *SEE ALSO:* health service area

service, aeromedical
SEE: aeromedical service

service assessment program (SAP)

service benefits
Insurance benefits paid in the form of health care services rather than cash.
SEE ALSO: indemnity benefits

service, central
SEE: central service

service charge, daily
SEE: daily service charge

service, chief of
SEE: chief of service

service, clinical
SEE: clinical service

service corporation
A nonprofit health benefit organization established for the purpose of providing coverage to individuals and groups, such as the Blue Cross and Blue Shield plans.

service corporation, dental
SEE: dental service corporation

service day, inpatient
SEE: inpatient service day

service, detoxification
SEE: detoxification service

service filtering
Referral of a patient to another provider or facility for services that are delivered at or below threshold levels.

service group, affiliated
SEE: affiliated service group

service, health care
SEE: health care service

service, home health
SEE: home health care

service industry weights (SIW)

service, professional
SEE: professional service

service recovery
Activities intended to address patient complaints and dissatisfaction.

services, community-based
SEE: community-based services

services, covered
SEE: covered services

services day, resident
SEE: resident services day

services, diagnostic
SEE: diagnostic services

services, emergency medical
SEE: emergency medical services

services, hospital-based
SEE: hospital-based services

service, social
SEE: social services

services, psychosocial
SEE: psychosocial services

services, referenced diagnostic
SEE: referenced diagnostic services

services, required
SEE: mandated services

services, supplemental
SEE: supplemental services

services, therapeutic
   SEE: therapeutic services

services, volunteer
   SEE: volunteer services

settlement, lump sum
   SEE: lump sum settlement

severity of illness
   The acuity of a patient's condition, based on clinical assessment.

SH
   social history

shadow pricing
   The practice of setting of insurance premium rates slightly below a competitor's rates.

shared housing
   A group home in which expenses and chores are shared among residents, who tend to be able-bodied persons interested in a community setting without the trouble of maintaining a single-family home.
   SYN: matched housing

shared risk pool
   A group of high-risk employers unable to obtain or afford insurance in the commercial marketplace who are equitably assigned to insurance companies for coverage, or who go into an assigned-risk pool operated by a state.
   SEE ALSO: residual market

share, market
   SEE: market share

sheltered living
   SEE: assisted living facility

shiatsu
   A traditional Japanese massage typically performed with the fingers that emphasizes healing by touching a network of pressure points on the body.

SHMO
social health maintenance organization

short-stay patient
A patient who occupies a hospital bed for a relatively short period, generally 24 hours or less, such as following minor surgery.
SYN: limited-stay patient

short-stay surgery
SEE: ambulatory surgery

short-term disability (STD)
A period of incapacitation, generally lasting six months or less.
SEE ALSO: long-term disability

SHP
state health plan

SHPDA
state health planning and development agency

SHPM
Society for Healthcare Planning and Marketing

SIA
Self-Insurance Institute of America

SIC
standard industrial code

sick baby
A newborn delivered with complications other than those related to prematurity.

SICU
surgical intensive care unit

side effect
An undesirable and unintentional result of medication or other therapy, usually considered, but is not always, harmful.
SEE ALSO: untoward effect

Sig
Instruction to patient

sign
An objective indication of disease or injury, which may be discovered by physical examination of the patient.
SEE ALSO: symptom

significant procedure
A procedure, usually scheduled, that is the primary reason for the patient's visit.

signs, vital
SEE: vital signs

similarly sized subscriber group (SSSG)

single carrier replacement
The coverage of an entire eligible group by one insurer and the discontinuation of all other health benefit plans.

single-payer system
A system of financing in which a single, centralized government entity pays for all health care costs, such as in Canada, Britain and Germany.

SIW
service industry weights

skilled nursing facility (SNF)
An inpatient facility that provides services for patients who are not acutely ill but require continuous health care.
SEE ALSO: subacute care

skimming
The practice of targeting low-risk individuals for enrollment by insurers and managed care plans and avoiding those who are more likely to have health problems and need more medical services.
SYN: cherry-picking

SLE
systemic lupus erythematosus

sliding fee scale
A method of charging for services on the basis of the patient's income and ability to pay.

SM
sports medicine

SMA
sequential multiple analyzer

SMI
supplemental medical insurance

SMSA
standard metropolitan statistical area

SNF
skilled nursing facility

SOAP
subjective, objective, assessment and plan.

SOB
shortness of breath

social health maintenance organization (SHMO)
A system to provide coordinated acute and long-term care for Medicare beneficiaries, typically including prescriptions and skilled nursing services.

social work, medical
SEE: medical social work

soft tissue
Skin and muscle.

sole proprietorship
A company owned by one individual.
SEE ALSO: corporation
partnership

sole-source option
An arrangement in which one insurer or managed care company covers all employees of a company, becoming a single source for all health care. Typically has an option for out-of-network services, with a greater share of the cost borne by the patient.

solo practice
A physician who operates alone, or with others, but keeps income and expenses separated.

somatoemotional release
An alternative medical approach believed to address the emotional impact of physical injury.

SPBA
Society of Professional Benefit Administrators

SPD
summary plan description

specialist
A physician or other health care provider whose training and expertise are in a specific area of medicine, such as neurology or cardiology. In managed care plans with a gatekeeper system, patients must see their primary care provider for referral to a specialist.

specialist, referral
SEE: referral specialist

specialty
A subject area or branch of medicine in which a health professional has particular education, training and expertise.

specialty care
Health services provided by a medical specialist, as opposed to primary care.
SYN: secondary care

SPECT
single photon emission computed tomography

speech therapy
The treatment of disorders affecting normal speech by a professional trained in speech pathology.

SpGr
specific gravity

spinal tap
> *SEE*: lumbar puncture

spin-off
> The voluntary sale or exchange of a subsidiary by a corporation.
> *SEE ALSO*: divestiture

spousal abuse
> The intentional emotional or physical mistreatment of a spouse or partner.

SSI
> Social Security Income Supplement

SSO
> second surgical opinion

SSOP
> second surgical opinion program

SSSG
> similarly sized subscriber group

staff, chief of
> *SEE*: chief of staff

staff, closed
> *SEE*: closed staff

staff, health care
> *SEE*: health care staff

staffing standards
> Guidelines for the number and type of health professionals needed to care for a population of patients, such as the number of physicians per 1,000 patients.

staff model
> A type of health maintenance organization in which physicians and other providers are employees of the company rather than independent contractors.
> *SEE ALSO*: health maintenance organization

staff model HMO
> *SEE*: closed panel

staff, open
> *SEE*: open staff

staff, visiting
> *SEE*: visiting staff

staging, disease
> *SEE*: disease staging

stain
1. Discoloration.
2. A dye used for the microscopic study of tissue or bacteria.
3. The process by which specimens are prepared with dye for microscopic study.

Standard benefit package
> *SEE*: basic benefit package

standard class rate (SCR)

standard industry code (SIC)

standard of care
The minimum acceptable patient care, based on statutes, court decisions, policies, or professional guidelines.
> *SEE ALSO*: negligence

standards, staffing
> *SEE*: staffing standards

stat
A designation commonly used by medical personnel indicating that a test or procedure is to be performed immediately.

statistical utilization review (SUR)

status, discharge
> *SEE*: discharge status

stay outlier
A patient whose hospitalization is significantly longer than other patients with a similar condition.
> *SYN*: day outlier

stay, days of
> SEE: length of stay

STD
> 1. sexually transmitted disease
> 2. short-term disability

steering
> The presence of financial incentives, such as lower out-of-pockets, to encourage a group of beneficiaries to seek medical care from a contracted network of providers.

step-down unit (SDU)

step therapy
> A regimen of drugs administered in sequence, often to control costs by using the least expensive drugs first.

sterilization
> 1. A procedure by which a person is rendered incapable of reproduction.
> 2. The elimination of all microorganisms on an object, such as by chemicals or pressurized steam.
> SEE ALSO: disinfection

stock acquisition
> The creation of a subsidiary by the purchase of majority voting interest in a company.
> SEE ALSO: stock acquisition

stop-loss
> An insurance contract that gives financial coverage above the point when expenses reach specified target levels.
> SYN: excess-loss
> excess-of-loss
> reinsurance
> risk control

stop-loss, aggregate
> SEE: aggregate stop-loss

stop-loss, individual
> SEE: individual stop-loss

stop-loss insurance
    SEE: reinsurance

stop-loss limit
    The dollar amount at which the reimbursement level of a health benefit plan increases to 100%, limiting the amount paid out-of-pocket by the covered individual.

structural integration
    SEE: rolfing

study, cohort
    SEE: cohort study

subacute care
    A comprehensive inpatient program for patients with serious illness or injury who do not require intensive hospital services. The range of services delivered in the subacute setting may include infusion therapy, respiratory therapy, rehabilitation, and postoperative recovery.

subcapitation
    An arrangement to carve out or subcontract certain services to another provider, and reimburse them by using a fraction of a total capitation payment per member per month.

subcutaneous
    Beneath the skin; a method of administering medications by injection.
    SYN: sub-q

subjective
    Based on opinion or judgment rather than an objective measurement.

subliminal therapy
    A form of self-help in which suggestions are delivered by subtle audio or visual means.

sub-q
    subcutaneous, or beneath the skin.

subrogation
A provision in some insurance policies requiring the insured individual to assign rights to recover damages to the insurer.

subscriber
A person who contracts for benefits with a health maintenance organization or other managed care plan. One subscriber can represent several enrollees, such as dependents that are included within a family benefit coverage .
SYN: beneficiary
SEE ALSO: enrollee
  member

subscriber, direct payment
SEE: direct payment subscriber

subspecialty
A narrowly focused area of practice within a clinical specialty, requiring additional training and expertise. For example, pediatric gastroenterology, the treatment of digestive conditions among child patients, is a subspecialty of pediatrics.
SYN: clinical subspecialty
SEE ALSO: specialty

substandard health insurance
An individual health insurance policy issued to a person who is unable to meet the minimum health requirements of a standard policy. May include waivers or additional premiums.
SEE ALSO: waiver

substantial comorbidity
SEE: comorbidity

succession of care
Maintenance of continuity of care during transfer of a patient from one health service or facility to another.
SEE ALSO: continuity of care

sugar pill
SEE: placebo

summary, benefit plan
SEE: benefit plan summary

summary plan description
    SEE: benefit plan summary

supplemental health insurance
    A policy covering medical expenses not included in a health plan held by an individual.
    SYN: wraparound

supplemental health services
    Health benefits offered by a health maintenance organization in excess of the minimum required under federal law.

supplemental medical insurance (SMI)

supplemental services
    Optional services that may be available for coverage in addition to basic health benefits, such as chiropractic, podiatric, dental or vision care.

support services, health care
    SEE: health care support services

SUR
    statistical utilization review

surcharge
    SEE: copayment

surgeon
    A physician who specializes in the treatment of diseases and conditions that require a surgical operation, rather than those primarily treated with drugs or some other noninvasive means. Literally, a physician who works with the hands.

surgery
    The treatment of injury or disease through an operative procedure, rather than by medication.

surgery, ambulatory
    SEE: ambulatory surgery

surgery, closed
    SEE: closed surgery

surgery, colon and rectal
 SEE: colon and rectal surgery

surgery, come-and-go
 SEE: ambulatory surgery

surgery, cosmetic
 SEE: cosmetic surgery

surgery, day
 SEE: ambulatory care facility

surgery, elective
 SEE: elective surgery

surgery, emergency
 SEE: emergency surgery

surgery, endoscopic
 SEE: endoscopic surgery

surgery, laparoscopic
 SEE: laparoscopic surgery

surgery, minimally invasive
 SEE: minimally invasive surgery

surgery, one-day
 SEE: ambulatory surgery

surgery, outpatient
 SEE: ambulatory surgery

surgery, short-stay
 SEE: ambulatory surgery

surgery, thoracic
 SEE: thoracic surgery

surgery, 23-hour
 SEE: ambulatory surgery

surgical expense insurance
 An insurance policy that provides coverage for physician or surgeon's fees related to an operation. Reimbursement may be determined by a surgical schedule.
 SEE ALSO: surgical schedule

surgical fee schedule
 SEE: surgical schedule

surgical schedule
 A list of fees attached to an insurance policy describing the maximum amount paid for specific surgical procedures.
 SYN: surgical fee schedule
 SEE ALSO: maximum allowable charges

surgicenter
 An independent, freestanding outpatient facility for surgical procedures that do not require hospitalization. May be affiliated with a hospital or privately owned.
 SYN: freestanding surgical center
 SEE ALSO: ambulatory care center

SV
 stroke volume

Swedish massage
 A vigorous massage intended to increase circulation and invigorate the body.

swing-bed hospital
 A rural hospital with fewer than 100 beds participating in a Medicare program that allows post-acute care services to be rendered in acute-care beds.

swing beds
 Hospital beds in an acute-care setting that may be used for long-term care.

SX
 symptoms

symptom
 A subjective phenomenon, physical impairment, or disruption of normal structure or function reported by a patient which suggests a disease or injury.

syndrome
 A number of associated signs and symptoms which together suggest a disease process.
 SEE ALSO: disease

system
1. An arrangement of tissues and organs which collectively perform specific body functions, such as respiration or metabolism.
2. An organization of personnel, facilities, and mechanisms that act in coordination for a specific purpose, such as an emergency medical service system.
3. A corporate body that owns or manages health care facilities and other related operations.

system abuse
The inappropriate utilization of health services, such as calling the 9-1-1 emergency number for transport to a hospital when no emergency exists and an alternate means of transportation is available.

system, gatekeeper
SEE: gatekeeper system

system, health
SEE: health system

system, health care
SEE: health care system

system, integrated delivery
SEE: integrated delivery system

system, single-payor
SEE: single-payor system

systemic
Referring to a condition that affects the whole body rather than an isolated area or part.
SEE ALSO: localized

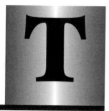

T
temperature

T&A
tonsillectomy and adenoidectomy

tab
tablet

TAB
therapeutic abortion

table rates
SEE: age-sex rates

table rating
SEE: age-sex rating

Tax Equity and Fiscal Responsibility Act of 1982 (TEFRA)
A federal law requiring employers to offer employees over the age of 65 the same health benefit plan as those under 65, in effect designating the employer as the primary insurer and Medicare as the secondary insurer.

tax preference
Laws that make the cost of health benefits paid by employers tax-deductible and not taxable for the employee.

TB
tuberculosis

teaching hospital
A medical center with a graduate medical education program, in which medical students, residents and other allied health professionals receive training.

technician, histologic
> *SEE:* histologic technician

technologist, circulation
> *SEE:* cardiovascular perfusionist

technologist, histologic
> *SEE:* histotechnologist

technology, adaptive
> *SEE:* adaptive technology

TEDS
> thrombo-embolytic disease stockings

TEE
> transesophageal echocardiogram

TEFRA
> Tax Equity and Fiscal Responsibility Act of 1982

tentative diagnosis
> *SEE:* admission diagnosis

terminal care document
> *SEE:* living will

term neonate
> An infant born within 39 to 42 weeks of gestation.

tertiary care
> Health care services that tend to be complex and sophisticated, usually more invasive and more reliant upon technology. Often has an affiliation with a medical school or teaching hospital.
> *SEE ALSO:* primary care
> secondary care

tertiary care facility
> A hospital that treats patients with complex conditions who are usually referred by other hospitals or specialist physicians.

tertiary prevention
> Medical interventions intended to prevent deterioration or the development of complications of a disease.

test
1. A determination of the presence (or absence) of a disease, a sign, or a substance in a body fluid or tissue.
2. A trial or evaluation period.

test, auxiliary
> *SEE:* auxiliary test

testing, preadmission
> *SEE:* preadmission testing

therapeutic
> A process, procedure or drug intended to alleviate a patient's illness or condition.

therapeutics
> The branch of medicine concerned with the treatment of illness or injury.
> *SYN:* therapy

therapeutic touch
> An alternative remedy in which a beneficial effect is believed to result from placing the hands on or near the patient's body.

therapist
> A person trained to treat illness or injury.

therapy
> The treatment of disease or injury.

therapy, art
> *SEE:* art therapy

therapy, cellular
> *SEE:* live cell therapy

therapy, chelation
> *SEE:* chelation therapy

therapy, colon
> *SEE:* colon therapy

therapy, color
> *SEE:* color therapy

therapy, drama
>   *SEE:* drama therapy

therapy, Gerson
>   *SEE:* Gerson therapy

therapy, Hoxey
>   *SEE:* Hoxey therapy

therapy, occupational
>   *SEE:* occupational therapy

therapy, physical
>   *SEE:* physical therapy

therapy, speech
>   *SEE:* speech therapy

therapy, step
>   *SEE:* step therapy

therapy, x-ray
>   *SEE:* radiation therapy

third-generation PPO
>   A PPO that employs case management, individual provider pro-
>   files, physician practice pattern analysis, and outcomes-based
>   quality measurement.

third-party administrator (TPA)
>   An organization that processes claims and pays providers for
>   self-insured groups or health maintenance organizations
>   (HMOs).

third-party agreement
>   An agreement that provides for payment of health care services
>   by someone other than the patient, such as an insurer, HMO,
>   employer or government.

third-party liability (TPL)
>   A third-party payer that is responsible for the cost of illness or
>   injury, such as an automobile insurance carrier.

third-party payer
1. An insurance company or health maintenance organization (HMO) plan.
2. A public or private organization that pays the health care bills of covered beneficiaries.
  SYN: carrier
     insurer

third-party payment
Payment for health services by an entity other than the patient, such as an insurer or government.

third-party reimbursement
A benefit program in which health services are paid by an entity other than the patient, i.e., an insurance company, government or self-insured employer.

thoracic surgeon
A physician who specializes in the surgical management of persons with disease or injury to structures of the chest.

thoracic surgery
1. Medical specialty involved in the diagnosis and treatment of disease or injury of the chest, including the lungs, heart and blood vessels.
2. Surgery of the chest.

threshold
1. Defined level at which an event or intervention is performed, or a focused review of medical care is conducted.
2. Upper and lower limits of perception, such as of sound or pain.

TIA
transient ischemic attack

t.i.d.
three times a day

tissue
Collection of similar cells.

tissue salts
>   *SEE:* Schuessler cell salts

Title XIX
>   Section of the federal Social Security Act that describes Medicaid services for the medically indigent.

Title XVIII
>   Section of the federal Social Security Act that describes Medicare coverage for the aged, blind and disabled.

TM
>   tympanic membrane

token payment
>   Modest amount of money, such as $1, paid by individuals for health care goods or services. Intended to limit utilization of health services. A feature sometimes found in comprehensive prepaid health plans.
>   *SYN:* hesitation payment
>   *SEE ALSO:* copayment
>   nominal payment

tomography, computed axial
>   *SEE:* computed axial tomography

tomography, positron emission
>   *SEE:* positron emission tomography

total budget
>   *SEE:* global budget

total charges
>   The sum of all charges for procedures, goods and services delivered by a provider in an encounter with the patient.

total disability
>   A condition that prevents a person from performing all work duties.
>   *SEE ALSO:* partial disability

total quality
An ongoing process to improve activities, products or services within an organization.

total quality management (TQM)

TPA
1. third-party administrator
2. tissue plasminogen activator

TPL
third-party liability

TPR
temperature, pulse, respiration

TQM
total quality management

TR
1. treatment
2. therapeutic radiology

traditional fee-for-service
The payment of health care services by a third-party payer or government.

training, in-service
SEE: in-service training

transfer
The movement of a patient from one hospital, inpatient unit, treatment facility or service to another.

transfer, inter-hospital
SEE: inter-hospital transfer

transplant
1. The surgical grafting of tissue or organs.
2. The tissue or organ that is surgically grafted.
SEE ALSO: allograft
homograft

trauma
Physical or emotional injury.

treatment
Surgical or medical management of a patient.
SEE ALSO: therapeutics
therapy

treatment algorithm
SEE: treatment protocol

treatment guideline
SEE: treatment protocol

treatment, least expensive alternate
SEE: least expensive alternative treatment

treatment, necessary
SEE: medically necessary

treatment plan
Proposed plan of treatment submitted by a provider to certify a patient for health benefits.

treatment protocol
Written guidelines for the medical treatment of patients with specific conditions. As strategies for patient management, treatment protocols assist physicians in clinical decision-making.
Syn: clinical pathway
cookbook medicine
medical practice plan
practice guideline
practice parameter
practice policies
treatment algorithm
treatment guideline

trend
Patterns or changes in data over a period of time.

trend factor
Conditions that influence the rate of change of medical costs, such as inflation, changes in utilization, cost-shifting and improvements in medical technology.

trending
Evaluation of patterns of data collected over a period of time.

triage
Process by which patients are categorized on the basis of the severity of illness or injury to determine the priority of treatment.

trial, clinical
SEE: clinical trial

trim points
Minimum and maximum length of hospital days for a diagnosis-related group (DRG). Patients whose hospitalization is more or less than the trim points are outliers.
SEE ALSO: outlier

triple option
Health benefit design that gives eligible individuals a choice of coverage under a health maintenance organization (HMO), a preferred provider organization (PPO) or traditional indemnity benefits. The costs of benefits and the share carried by the beneficiary vary among the types of plans.

TRS
trauma surgery

trust, multiple employer
SEE: multiple employer trust

TS
thoracic surgery

TSH
thyroid-stimulating hormone

TURP
transurethral resection of the prostate

TV
tidal volume

TX
1. traction
2. treatment

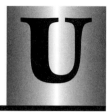

U
1. urology
2. urological surgery

UA
urinalysis

UB-92
Claim form commonly used by medical facilities to bill for health care services and products.

UC
usual, customary, and reasonable fees

UCHD
usual childhood diseases

UCR
usual, customary, and reasonable charges

UEHB
uniform effective health benefits

UHDDS
uniform hospital discharge data set

ultrasound
Noninvasive means of imaging organs and other internal structures of the body with high-frequency sound waves.

UM
1. utilization management
2. underseas medicine

UMC
utilization management coordinator

unallocated benefit

Health insurance provision specifying reimbursement up to a maximum amount for all extra or miscellaneous hospital services without specifying limits for each type of service.

SEE ALSO: allocated benefit

unbundling

Practice of breaking down a procedure or process into separate billable charges for the purpose of increasing reimbursement under a health benefit plan.

SYN: fragmentation

SEE ALSO: gaming the system

uncompensated care

Health care services that are not paid by the patient or a third-party payer.

SEE ALSO: unsponsored care

underinsurance

SEE: medically indigent

underwriting

Process of evaluating and classifying the degree of financial risk represented by a pool of proposed insured individuals.

uniform effective health benefits (UEHB)

uniform hospital discharge data set (UHDDS)

uninsured

SEE: medically indigent

unintentional injury

Anatomic or functional impairment as a result of unexpected trauma.

SYN: accident

unit, burn

SEE: burn unit

unit clerk

Person who assists with administrative and support tasks in an inpatient unit, including answering telephones, processing pa-

perwork, transcribing orders, scheduling appointments, ordering supplies, updating medical records and other duties.
SYN: ward clerk

unit, live-in
SEE: live-in unit

unit manager
Administrator of a medical or nursing unit in a health care facility.
SYN: ward manager

unit, step-down
SEE: step-down unit

universal precautions
Guidelines established by the federal Centers for Disease Control for preventing the spread of infectious disease, including the use of gloves, masks, gowns and other barriers.

unmanaged care
1. Health care services not subject to cost, quality or utilization controls.
2. Traditional fee-for-service reimbursement.
SEE ALSO: fee-for-service
managed care

unnecessary care
Medical services that are not indicated by the patient's condition, treatment guidelines, or the current standard of care.

unnecessary stays
Admissions to hospitals that are determined by a health plan to be inappropriate for the nature of the patients' medical condition.

unremarkable
Not significant or worthy of noting.

unrestricted funds
Money that has no conditions placed on its expenditure, and therefore may be applied to any legitimate need.
SEE ALSO: restricted funds

unsponsored care
Total cost of services provided to patients for which payment is not received, a sum of bad-debt and charity care.
SYN: uncompensated care
SEE ALSO: bad debt
charity care
medically indigent

untoward effect
Potentially harmful and undesired result of medication or other therapy.
SEE ALSO: side effect

upcoding
Practice of billing a health benefit plan for a procedure that reimburses the provider at a greater rate than the procedure actually performed.
SYN: code creep
SEE ALSO: gaming the system
overcoding

UR
utilization review

URAC
Utilization Review Accreditation Commission

URC
utilization review coordinator

urgent admission
Patient who requires hospitalization for the immediate care of illness or injury.
SYN: emergency admission

urgent care
Treatment of injuries or conditions that require prompt medical attention in order to prevent serious deterioration of a patient's health, but are not life threatening.
SEE ALSO: emergency

urgent care center
Facility for the treatment of conditions or injuries that require immediate medical attention, but are not life threatening.

URI
upper respiratory infection

urine therapy
Unconventional remedy in which a person's own urine is taken for therapeutic purposes.

URO
utilization review organization

USP
United States Pharmacopeia

usual fee
Fee that a provider most often charges for a specific procedure or health care service.
SEE ALSO: customary fee
prevailing fee
reasonable fee

usual, customary and reasonable fees (UCR)
Insurance industry term referring to the normal, prevailing charges in a community, state or region that will be reimbursed by an insurer or health maintenance organization (HMO) plan.
SEE ALSO: maximum allowable charges

USUHS
Uniformed Services University of the Health Sciences

UTI
u294rinary tract infection

utilization
1. Consumption of health care goods or services.
2. Level of medical services used by a defined population within a specific time period.

utilization management (UM)
Review and moderation of the consumption of health care services and resources. Generally includes systems to monitor the use of services, authorization for specialty care and hospitalization, and other strategies to ensure that care is appropriate and cost-effective.
SEE ALSO: managed care

utilization rate
Amount of health care services used by a group of patients within a period of time, usually expressed as units of service per year per 1,000 eligible individuals.

utilization review (UR)
Formal assessment of the cost and use of components of the health care system.
SEE ALSO: concurrent review
managed care
retrospective review
utilization management

utilization review organization (URO)
Company that provides utilization review for managed care organizations.

utilization review, statistical
SEE: statistical utilization review

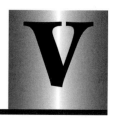

VA
Veterans Administration

validation criteria
Objective health care standards used to determine whether the diagnosis or condition of a patient is accurately reflected in the medical record.
SEE ALSO: combined audit
concurrent review
retrospective review
utilization review

validation criterion
Determination whether a patient had the condition described as the diagnosis in the medical record.

validity
Degree to which an indicator or other factor accurately reflects a state or event.
SEE ALSO: reliability

VAMC
Veterans Administration Medical Center

variable costs
Expenses that change depending on the volume or level of activity
SEE ALSO: fixed costs
semivariable costs

variance analysis
Assessment of actual results compared to expected results.
SYN: variation analysis

variance report
Document categorizing medical records based on conformation to validation criteria.
SEE ALSO: validation criteria

variation
1. Discrepancy between screening criteria and information contained in a medical record.
2. Difference between expected and actual results.
SEE ALSO: screening criteria
variation analysis

variation record
Patient record that fails to comply with criteria employed in an audit.

vascular
Pertaining to blood vessels.

VC
vital capacity

VCU
voiding cystourethrogram

VEBA
Voluntary Employees' Beneficiary Association

venture, joint
SEE: joint venture

vertical integration
Organization of different types of providers who together offer a comprehensive range of providers, such as a system consisting of outpatient primary care, inpatient hospital care, and long-term convalescent care.
SEE ALSO: horizontal integration

viability
Capable of living.

viatical settlement
SYN: viatication
SEE ALSO: accelerated death benefit

viatication
> *Syn:* viatical settlement
> *See:* accelerated death benefit

virulence
Capacity of a micro-organism to produce illness.

visiting staff
Physicians, nurse practitioners, therapists and other allied personnel in private practice who are authorized to use the facilities of a hospital to care for their patients.

visualization
> *See:* imagery

vital signs
Measures of body function used to assess the status of the patient, including temperature, pulse rate, respiratory rate and blood pressure.

vitamin therapy
The use of vitamins, minerals and other nutritional supplements for therapeutic purposes.

vocational rehabilitation
A therapeutic program intended to help the person recovering from severe illness or injury to cope with the physical and emotional demands of employment.

volume performance standards (VPS)

voluntary employees' beneficiary association (VEBA)
Organization that provides a means for a group of employees to create a tax-free reserve for the provision of health, life, disability or other benefits.
> *Syn:* 501(c)(9) trust

voluntary enrollment
Selection of a managed care plan from two or more options, such as when an employer offers a number of health benefit plans.

voluntary hospital
Non-profit, tax-exempt hospital which has a mission to provide benefits to the community in which it operates.
SEE ALSO: community benefits

volunteer
Person who donates his or her time to work in a health care facility.
SYN: candystriper
SEE ALSO: hospital auxiliary
pink ladies

volunteer, in-service
SEE: in-service volunteer

volunteer services
Services performed by non-paid individuals who donate their time to health care facilities. Volunteers typically perform non-medical duties, such as answering telephones, escorting patients and families, operating gift shop or dining area.
SEE ALSO: candystriper
hospital auxiliary
pink ladies

VPS
volume performance standards

VS
1. vascular surgery
2. vital signs

VSD
ventricular septal defect

vulnerable adults
Persons who are unable to meet their own needs due to physical or mental conditions.

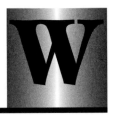

wa
while awake

waiting list
Roster of patients in line for access to a hospital, nursing home or other health facility or service.

waiting period
1. Period of time following enrollment in a health benefit plan in which pre-existing conditions are not covered.
2. Duration between a work-related injury and the commencement of disability compensation.

waiver
Provision of a health benefit contract specifically excluding certain conditions from coverage.
SYN: exception
exclusion

waiver of premium
Provision in a health benefit contract in which the insured does not have to pay the premium while he or she is disabled.

walker
Tubular frame constructed of sturdy yet lightweight material used to assist persons with walking.

wanton negligence
Deliberate and conscious action or inaction that exhibits reckless disregard for the consequences and that could cause injury.
SEE ALSO: malpractice
negligence

ward
1. Guardianship of a person who is unable to care for himself or herself. Often the individual is a child, and generally guardianship is ordered by a court.
2. Hospital room with three or more beds.

ward clerk
SEE: unit clerk

ward manager
SEE: unit manager

ward patients
Medically indigent patients who are treated at a public or teaching hospital.

water pill
Informal term for a diuretic, a medication that increases the output of the kidneys.
SYN: diuretic

WBC
1. white blood cell
2. white blood count

WBGH
Washington Business Group on Health

WDC
weighted daily census

WDWN
well-developed and well-nourished

weekend hospital
Facility for the partial hospitalization of patients, who may spend weekdays in the community and weekends at the facility.
SEE ALSO: partial hospitalization

weight, birth
SEE: birth weight

weighted daily census (WDC)

weighting
Assignment of greater value to a factor or variable. Under the RBRVS system, the fee for a service may be weighted depending on the number of times it is charged.

well-baby care
Routine examinations, immunizations and other medical services considered routine for a healthy infant.

wellness
Philosophy and health care approach that promotes fitness, healthful lifestyles, early detection of disease and preventive medicine.

well newborn
Healthy, full-term infant born under controlled conditions in a hospital.

WHEA
Women's Health Equity Act

wheelchair
Specialized mobility device for use by disabled persons.

WHO
World Health Organization

wholesale price, average
SEE: average wholesale price

willful negligence
Intentional omission or commission of a duty or act of proper care that disregards the safety, health, life or rights of another person.
SEE ALSO: malpractice

withhold
Portion of physician compensation held by a managed care organization, and returned to the providers if the utilization of health services by patients is below specified levels. The withhold becomes permanent if utilization and/or costs exceed targets.
SYN: physician contingency reserve

withhold pool
Amount of money retained from capitated payments or discounted fees to primary care physicians or specialists and held to incentivize physicians to manage utilization and costs and eliminate excessive health care expenditures.
SYN: risk pool
SEE ALSO: at-risk contracting

wk
week

WNL
within normal limits

Women's Health Equity Act (WHEA)

workers' comp
SEE: workers' compensation

workers' compensation
System established by statutes in each state to provide benefits to individuals who experience work-related injury, illness or death.
SYN: workers' comp

workers' compensation insurance
Insurance policy that provides health care coverage and disability payments for work-related illness or injury.

work hardening
Program of physical conditioning, workplace modifications and other interventions intended to help a disabled person return to gainful employment.
SEE ALSO: modified work duty

work-up
Evaluation of a patiént, including the history, physical examination, laboratory and radiological findings.
SYN: patient assessment

World Health Organization (WHO)

wraparound
  Supplemental benefit plan that pays for health costs not covered by a basic benefit plan, such as Medicare.

write-off
  Debt that cannot be collected and is deducted from gross revenue.
  Syn: bad debt

written authorization
  Document giving consent or permission for one person to act on behalf of another.

written premium
  Total amount charged over a period of a year for health benefits specified in a contract.

wrongful death
  1. Mortality of a patient due to an error in the course of medical care.
  2. Death of any individual caused or thought to be caused by negligence on the part of some party.
  3. Lawsuit filed by surviving family members of a deceased patient against those who are responsible for the death.

Wt
  weight

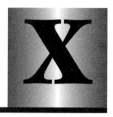

X-ray
1. High-energy electromagnetic radiation produced by striking a target with a beam of electrons in a vacuum tube.
2. Production of an image of bone and other internal structures for the purpose of assessing a patient's condition.
   SYN: Roentgen ray

X-ray therapy
Use of radiation in the treatment of disease.
   SYN: radiation therapy
   SEE ALSO: nuclear medicine

xenograft
Transplantation of tissue taken from a donor other than the patient.

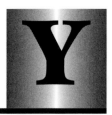

yo
   years old

yr
   year

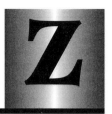

ZEBRA
zero balanced reimbursement account

zero balanced reimbursement account (ZEBRA)
Health benefit plan used by self-insured employers which pays for health services as it is rendered.
SYN: cafeteria plan

zone therapy
SEE: reflexology

zoonosis
Transmission of infectious disease between animals and humans.
SYN: zoonotic disease

zoonotic disease
SEE: zoonosis

BIBLIOGRAPHIC REFERENCES

BOOKS

Accreditation Manual for Hospitals, Volume 1. Chicago: Joint Commission for the Accreditation of Healthcare Organizations, 1995.

Berman HJ, Kukla SF. The Financial Management of Hospitals, 8th ed. Ann Arbor, MI: Health Administration Press, 1994.

Coders' Desk Reference. Salt Lake City: Medicode, 1995.

Fazen, MF. Managed Care Desk Reference: The Complete Guide to Terminology and Resources. Dallas: HCS Publications, 1994.

Glossary of Hospital and Health Care System Merger, Acquisition, and Consolidation Terms. Chicago: American Hospital Association, 1989.

Handel B, ed. Glossary of Health Care Terms, 2nd ed. Brookfield, WI: International Foundation of Employee Benefit Plans, 1991.

Hanken MA, Water KA, eds. Glossary of Healthcare Terms. Chicago: American Health Information Management Association, 1994.

Hogue K. The Complete Guide to Health Insurance. New York: Walker Publishing, 1988.

Nathanson MD. Home Health Care Answer Book. Gaithersburg, MD: Aspen, 1995.

O'Leary MR. Lexikon: Dictionary of Health Care Terms, Organizations, and Acronyms for the Era of Reform. Oakbrook Terrace, IL: Joint Commission on Accreditation of Healthcare Organizations, 1994.

Restructuring Health Care Delivery—Legal and Common Terms. Chicago: American Hospital Association, 1994.

Slee VN, Slee DA. Health Care Reform Terms, 2nd ed. St. Paul, MN: Tringa Press, 1994.

Slee VN, Slee DA. Health Care Terms, 2nd ed. St. Paul, MN: Tringa Press, 1991.

Source Book of Health Insurance Data. Washington, DC: Health Insurance Association of America, 1994. (no author)

Stedman's Medical Dictionary, 26th ed. Baltimore: Williams and Wilkins, 1995.

Timmreck TC. Dictionary of Health Services Management, 2nd ed. Owings Mills, MD: National Health Publishing, 1987.

Ward WJ, Jr. Health Care Budgeting and Financial Management for Non-Financial Managers. Westport, CT: Auburn House, 1994.

Willis MC. Medical Terminology. Baltimore: Williams and Wilkins, 1996.

PERIODICALS

Hartwell T, Hamilton BU. Managed care resource guide. Medical Group Management Journal 1994;41(5): 50–74.

WORLD WIDE WEB SITES

http://www.freenet.scri.fsu.edu/doc/flhp.doc24. Glossary section of the Florida Health Security Plan.

http://www.orst.edu/faculty/neilson/glossary. Glossary of insurance terms.

http://members.gnn.com/subacute/glossary.htm. Managed care and post-acute care glossary.

http://weber.u.washington.edu/ ~ larsson/hsic94/resource/glossary.html. Health care administration glossary of terms.

http://www.ada.org.prac/man-care/glossary.html. Managed care glossary, sponsored by the American Dental Association.

http://www-med.stanford.edu/MedCenter/SHS/primaryCare/primcare. glossary.html. Stanford primary care glossary.

http://www.cols-ceo.com/cols_ceo.gra/health/hc_40.html. Health systems terms.

http://ww.medsource.com/define.html. Key integration and managed care definitions.

http://www.crl.com/ ~ balbel/dict.htm. Dictionary of definitions and distinctions.

http://www.ncqa.org/glossary.htm. A glossary of managed care terms, sponsored by the National Commission for Quality Assurance.

http://www.tne/com/glossary/glossary.htm. Financial glossary.

http://www.cmhc.com/articles/glossary.htm. Managed care glossary, sponsored by Mental Health Net.

http://www.mahmo.org/hmoterms.html. Glossary of HMO-related terms, sponsored by the Massachusetts Association of HMOs.

COMMON ABBREVIATIONS AND SYMBOLS USED IN THE MEDICAL RECORD

$\overline{aa}$	of each
$\overline{a}$	before
Ⓑ	bilateral
$\overline{c}$	with
ⓜ	murmur
$\overline{p}$	after
$\overline{s}$	without
$\overline{ss}$	one-half
V_T	tidal volume
♀	female
♂	male
#	number or pound
°	degree or hour
↑	increased or above
↓	decreased or below
ϴ	none or negative
♀	standing
♀	sitting
○—	lying
×	times or for
>	greater than
<	less than
ꙓ	one
ꙓꙓ	two
ꙓꙓꙓ	three
ꙓ̄v	four
O_2	oxygen
PaO_2	arterial partial pressure of oxygen
$PaCO_2$	arterial partial pressure of carbon dioxide

APPENDIX 2
COMMON HEALTH CARE FORMULAS

$$\text{Average Daily Census} = \frac{\text{total number of patients}}{\text{days in time period under study}}$$

$$\text{Average Length of Stay} = \frac{\text{total length of hospitalization}}{\text{total discharges and deaths}}$$

Hospital Autopsy Rate =

$$\frac{\text{total number of autopsies} \times 100}{\text{number of patient deaths eligible for autopsy}}$$

Occupancy Ratio =

$$\frac{\text{total number of service days in study period} \times 100}{\text{total capacity during study period}}$$

Turnover Rate =

$$\frac{\text{total number of discharges in study period}}{\text{total capacity during study period}}$$

APPENDIX 3
PROFESSIONAL ORGANIZATIONS

Academy of Managed Care Pharmacy (AMCP)
1321 Duke St.,
Suite 305
Alexandria, VA 22314
703/683-8412
703/683-8417 fax

American Academy of Allergy and Immunology (AAAI)
611 E. Wells St.
Milwaukee, WI 53202
414/272-6071
414/276-3349 fax

American Academy of Ambulatory Care Nursing (AAACN)
Box 56, N. Woodbury Rd.
Pitman, NJ 08071
609/256-2350
609/589-7463 fax

American Academy of Dermatology (AAD)
930 N. Meacham Rd.
Schaumburg, IL 60172-4965
708/330-0230
708/330-0050 fax

American Academy of Family Physicians (AAFP)
8880 Ward Parkway
Kansas City, MO 64114
816/333-9700
816/822-0580 fax

American Academy of Neurology (AAN)
2221 University Ave. SE,
Suite 335
Minneapolis, MN 55414
612/623-8115
612/623-3504 fax

American Academy of Nurse Practitioners (AANP)
LBJ Building
P. O. Box 12846 Capital Station
Austin, TX 78711
512/442-4263
512/442-6468 fax

American Academy of Ophthalmology (AAO)
655 Beach St.
San Francisco, CA 94109
415/561-8511
415/561-8533 fax

American Academy of Orthopaedic Surgeons (AAOS)
6300 N. River Rd.
Rosemont, IL 60018-4226
708/823-7186
708/823-8125 fax

American Academy of Osteopathy (AAO)
3500 DePauw Blvd.,
Suite 1080
Indianapolis, IN 46248-1136
317/879-1881
317/879-0563 fax

American Academy of Pediatrics (AAP)
141 Northwest Point Blvd.
P.O. Box 927
Elk Grove Village IL 60009-0927
708/228-5005
708/228-5097 fax

American Academy of Physical Medicine and Rehabilitation (AAPMR)
1 IBM Plaza, 25th Floor
Chicago, IL 60611-3604
312-464-9700
312-464-0227

American Academy of Physician Executives (AAPE)
4890 W. Kennedy Blvd., Suite 200
Tampa, FL 33609
813/287-2000
813/287-8993 fax

American Association of Blood Banks (AABB)
8101 Glenbrook Rd.
Bethesda, MD 20814-2719
301/907-6977
301/907-6896 fax

American Association for Continuity of Care (AACC)
1720 N. Lynn St.
Arlington, VA 22209
703/525-1191
703/276-8196 fax

American Association of Healthcare Consultants (AAHC)
11208 Waples Mill Rd., Suite 109
Fairfax, VA 22030
703/691-2242

American Association of Health Plans (AAHP)
1129 20th St. NW, Suite 600
Washington, DC 20036
202/778-3200
202/331-7487 fax

American Association of Physician-Hospital Organizations (AAPHO)
P. O. Box 4913
Glen Allen, VA 23058
800/722-0376
804/747-5316 fax

American Association of Preferred Provider Organizations (AAPPO)
1101 Connecticut Ave. NW, Suite 700
Washington, DC 20036
202/429-5733
202/429-5108 fax

American Association for Medical Transcription (AAMT)
P. O. Box 57187
Modesto, CA 95357-6187
209/551-0883
209/551-9317 fax

American Association of Managed Care Nurses (AAMCN)
P. O. Box 4975
Glen Allen, VA 23058-4975
804/747-9698
804/747-5316 fax

American Board of Internal Medicine (ABIM)
3624 Market St.
Philadelphia, PA 19104
215/243-1500

American Board of Medical
Specialties (ABMS)
1007 Church St.,
Suite 404
Evanston, IL 60201-5913
708/491-9091
708/328-3596 fax

American Board of Preventive
Medicine (ABPM)
9950 W. Lawrence Ave.,
Suite 106
Schiller Park, IL 60176
708/671-1750
708/671-1751 fax

American Cancer Society
(ACS)
1599 Clifton Rd. NE
Atlanta, GA 30329
404/320-3333
404/325-0230 fax

American Chiropractic
Association (ACA)
1701 Clarendon Blvd.
Arlington, VA 22209
703/276-8800
703/243-2593 fax

American Clinical Laboratory
Association (ACLA)
1250 H St. NW, Suite 880
Washington, DC 20005
202/637-9466
202/637-2050 fax

American College of Chest
Physicians (ACCP)
3300 Old Georgetown Rd.
Bethesda, MD 20814-1699
301/897-5400
301/897-9745 fax

American College of Emergency
Physicians (ACEP)
P. O. Box 619911
Dallas, TX 75261-9911
214/550-0911
214/580-2816 fax

American College of Healthcare
Administrators (ACHA)
325 S. Patrick St.
Alexandria, VA 22314
703/549-5822
703/739-7901

American College of Healthcare
Executives (ACHE)
840 N. Lake Shore Dr. 1103W
Chicago, Il 60611
312/943-0544
312/943-3791

American College of Medical
Quality (ACMQ)
9005 Congressional Ct.
Potomac, MD 20854
301/365-3570
301/365-3202 fax

American College of
Obstetricians and
Gynecologists (ACOG)
409 12th St. NW
Washington, DC 20024
202/638-5577
202/484-8107 fax

American College of Physicians
(ACP)
Independence Mall West
6th St. at Race
Philadelphia, PA 91106
215/351-2400
215/351-2448 fax

American College of
Rheumatology (ACR)
60 Executive Park S,
Suite 150
Atlanta, GA 30329
404/633-3777
404/633-1870 fax

American College of Surgeons
(ACS)
55 E. Erie St.
Chicago, IL 60611
312/664-4050
312/440-7014 fax

American Dental Association
(ADA)
211 E. Chicago Ave.
Chicago, IL 60611
312/440-2500

American Diabetes Association
(ADA)
P. O. Box 25757
1660 Duke St.
Alexandria, VA 22314
703/549-1500
703/836-7439 fax

American Federation of Home
Health Agencies
(AFHHA)
1320 Fenwick Ln., Suite 100
Silver Spring, MD 20910
301/588-1454
301/588-4732 fax

American Group Practice
Association (AGPA)
1422 Duke St.
Alexandria, VA 22314-3430
703/838-0033
703/548-1890 fax

American Health Care
Association (AHCA)
1201 L St. NW
Washington, DC 20005-4014
202/842-4444
202/842-3860 fax

American Health Information
Management Association
(AHIMA)
919 N. Michigan Ave.,
Suite 1400
Chicago, IL 60611-1683
312/787-2672
312/787-9893 fax

American Heart Association
(AHA)
7272 Greenville Ave.
Dallas, TX 75231-4596
214/373-6300
214/706-1341

American Hospital Association
(AHA)
840 N. Lake Shore Dr.
Chicago, IL 60611
312/280-6000
312/280-5979 fax

American Medical Association
(AMA)
515 N. State St.
Chicago, IL 60610
312/464-5000
312/464-4184 fax

American Medical Peer Review
Association (AMPRA)
810 First St. NE, Suite 410
Washington, DC 20002
202/371-5610
202/371-8954 fax

American Nurses Association (ANA)
600 Maryland Ave. SW,
Suite 100W
Washington, DC 20021-2571
202/651-7000
202/651-7001 fax

American Osteopathic Healthcare Association (AOHA)
5301 Wisconsin Ave. NW,
Suite 630
Washington, DC 20015
202/686-1700
202/686-7615 fax

American Pharmaceutical Association (APA)
2215 Constitution Ave. NW
Washington, DC 20037
202/628-4410
202/783-2351

American Podiatric Medicine Association (APMA)
8312 Old Georgetown Rd.
Bethesda, MD 20814
301/571-9200
301/53-2752 fax

American Psychiatric Association (APA)
1400 K St. NW
Washington, DC 20005
202/682-6000
202/682-6114 fax

American Psychological Association (APA)
750 First St NE
Washington, DC 20002-4242
202/336-5500

American Public Health Association (APHA)
1015 15th St. NW
Washington, DC 20005
202/789-5600
202/789-5681 fax

American Rehabilitation Association (ARA)
1910 Association Drive, Suite 200
Reston, VA 22091
703/648-9300
703/648-0346 fax

American Society for Healthcare Risk Management (ASHRM)
840 N. Lake Shore Dr.
Chicago, IL 60611
312/280-6430
312/280-4151

American Society of Plastic and Reconstructive Surgeons (ASPRS)
444 E. Algonquin Rd.
Arlington Heights, IL 60005
708/228-9900
708/228-9131 fax

American Thoracic Society (ATA)
1740 Broadway
New York, NY 10019-4374
212/315-8700
212/315-6498 fax

American Urological Association (AUA)
1120 N. Charles St.
Baltimore, MD 21201
410/727-1100
410/625-2390 fax

Blue Cross and Blue Shield Association (BCBSA)
676 N. St. Clair St.
Chicago, IL 60611
312/440-6000
312/440-6609 fax

Case Management Society of America (CMSA)
1101 17th St. NW, Suite 1200
Washington, DC 20036
202/296-9200
202/296-0023 fax

Employee Assistance Professionals Association (EAPA)
4601 N. Fairfax Dr.,
Suite 1001
Arlington, VA 22203
703/522-6272
703/522-4585 fax

Federation of American Health Systems (FAHS)
1111 19th St NW,
Suite 402
Washington, DC 20036
202/833-3090
202/861-0063 fax

Health Insurance Association of America (HIAA)
1025 Connecticut Ave. NW
Washington, DC 20036-3998
202/223-7800
202/223-7897 fax

Hospice Association of America (HAA)
519 C St. NE
Washington, DC 20002
202/546-4759
202/547-3540 fax

Individual Case Management Association (ICMA)
10809 Executive Center Dr.,
Suite 105
Little Rock, AR 72211-6020
501/227-5553
501/227-8362

International Subacute Healthcare Association (ISHA)
4040 W. 70th St.
Minneapolis, MN 55435
612/926-1773
612/926-1624 fax

Joint Commission on the Accreditation of Healthcare Organization (JCAHO)
1 Renaissance Blvd.
Oak Brook, IL 60181
708/916-5600
708/916-5644 fax

Managed Health Care Association (MHCA)
1225 Eye St. NW, Suite 300
Washington, DC 20005
202/371-8232
202/842-0621 fax

Medical Group Management Association (MGMA)
104 Iverness Terrace E
Englewood, CO 80112
303/799-1111
303/643-4427 fax

Medical Records Institute (MRI)
P. O. Box 289
Newton, MA 02160
617/964-3923
617/964-3926 fax

National Association for
Ambulatory Care (NAAC)
21 Michigan St.
Grand Rapids, MI 49503
616/949-2138

National Association for
Healthcare Quality
(NAHQ)
5700 Old Orchard Rd., 1st Floor
Skokie, IL 60077
708/965-2776
708/966-9418 fax

National Association for Home
Care (NAHC)
519 C St. NE
Washington, DC 20002
202/547-7424
202/547-3540 fax

National Association of
Insurance Commissioners
(NAIC)
120 W. 12th St., Suite 1100
Kansas City, MO 64105
816/842-3600
816/471-7004 fax

National Association of
Managed Care Physicians
(NAMCP)
4435 Waterfront Dr., Suite 101
Glen Allen, VA 23060
804/527-1905
804/747-5316 fax

National Committee for Quality
Assurance (NCQA)
1350 New York Ave. NW,
Suite 700
Washington, DC 20005
202/628-5788
202/628-0344 fax

National Health Lawyers
Association (NHLA)
1620 Eye St. NW,
Suite 900
Washington, DC 20006
202/833-1100
202/833-1105 fax

National Mental Health
Association (NMHA)
1021 Prince St
Alexandria, VA 22314-2971
703/684-7722
703/684-5968 fax

National Rehabilitation
Association (NRA)
633 S. Washington St.
Alexandria, VA 22314
703/836-0850
703/836-0848 fax

National Rural Health
Association (NRHA)
301 E. Armour Blvd.,
Suite 420
Kansas City, MO 64111
816/756-3140
816/756-3144 fax

Risk and Insurance
Management Society
(RIMS)
205 E. 42nd St., 15th Floor
New York, NY 10017
212/286-9292
212/986-9716 fax

Self-Insurance Institute of
America (SIA)
P. O. Box 15466
Santa Ana, CA 93705
714/261-2553
714/261-2594 fax

Society for Healthcare Planning and Marketing (SHPM)
840 N. Lake Shore Dr.
Chicago, IL 60611
312/280-6086
312/280-6252 fax

Society of Critical Care Medicine (SCCM)
8101 E. Kaiser Blvd.
Anaheim, CA 92808
714/282-6000
714/282-6050 fax

Society of Professional Benefit Administrators (SPBA)
2 Wisconsin Circle, Suite 670
Chevy Chase, MD 20815-7003
301/718-7722
301/718-9440 fax

GOVERNMENT AGENCIES AND ADVISORY GROUPS

Agency for Health Care Policy and Research (AHCPR)
2102 E. Jefferson St., Suite 603
Rockville, MD 20852
301/227-8459
301/277-8157 fax

Centers for Disease Control and Prevention (CDC)
1600 Clifton Road NE
Atlanta, GA 30333
404/639-3311

Clinical Laboratory Improvement Advisory Committee (CLIAC)
Public Health Practice Program
Office S-E20
Centers for Disease Control and Prevention
1600 Clifton Road NE,
Mailstop G-25
Atlanta, GA 30333
404/639-1902

Department of Health and Human Services (DHHS)
200 Independence Ave., SW
Washington, DC 20201
202/619-0257

Food and Drug Administration (FDA)
5600 Fishers Lane
Parklawn Building
Rockville, MD 20857
301/443-1544

Health Care Financing Administration (HCFA)
200 Independence Ave, SW
Washington, DC 20001
202/690-6726

Health Resources and Services Administration (HRSA)
5600 Fishers Lane, Room 14-45
Parklawn Building
Rockville, MD 20857
301/443-2086
301/443-1989

National Advisory Committee on Rural Health (NACRH)
Office of Rural Health Policy
Health Resources and Services Administration
Parklawn Building, Room 9-05
5600 Fishers Lane
Rockville, MD 20857
301/443-0835
301/443-2805 fax

National Institutes of Health (NIH)
9000 Rockville Pike
Bethesda, MD 20892
301/496-4000

National Practitioner Data Bank (NPDB)
P. O. Box 6050
Camarillo, CA 93011
800/767-6732

Office of Prepaid Health Care Operations and Oversight (OPHCOO)
Cohen Building, Room 4406
330 Independence Avenue, SW
Washington, DC 20201
202/619-0845
202/619-2011 fax

Physician Payment Review Commission (PPRC)
2120 L Street NW, Suite 200
Washington, DC 20037
202/653-7220
202/653-7238 fax

Prospective Payment Assessment Commission (ProPAC)
300 7th St., SW, Suite 301B
Washington, DC 20024
202/401-8986
202/401-8739 fax

HEALTH POLICY AND RESEARCH GROUPS

Employee Benefits Research Institute (EBRI)
2121 K St. NW, Suite 600
Washington, DC 20037-1896
202/659-0670
202/775-6312 fax

Health Outcomes Institute (HOI)
2001 Killebrew Dr., Suite 122
Bloomington, MN 55425
612/858-9188
612/858-9189 fax

Interstudy
2901 Metro Dr.,
Suite 400
Bloomington, MN 55331
612/858-9291
612/854-5698 fax

National Managed Health Care Congress (NMHCC)
1000 Winter St., Suite 4000
Waltham, MA 02154
617/487-6700
617/487-6709 fax

Fobert Wood Johnson Foundation
College Road, P. O. Box 2316
Princeton, NJ 08543-2316
609/452-8701

Washington Business Group on Health (WBGH)
777 N. Capitol St, Suite 800
Washington, DC 20002
202/408-9392
202/408-9332 fax

Accreditation Association for Ambulatory Health Care (AAAHC)
9933 Lawler Ave.
Skokie, IL 60077-3708
708/676-6910
708/676-9628 fax

American Accreditation Program, Inc. (AAP)
2270 Cedar Cove Court
Reston, VA 22091
703/860-5900
703/860-5901 fax

Commission on Accreditation of Rehabilitation Facilities (CARF)
101 N. Wilmot Rd., Suite 500
Tucson, AZ 85711
602/748-1212

Joint Commission on Accreditation of Healthcare Organizations (JCAHO)
One Renaissance Blvd.
Oakbrook Terrace, IL 60181
708/916-5800
708/916-5644 fax

National Accrediting Agency for Clinical Laboratory Sciences (NAACLS)
8410 W. Bryn Mawr Ave.,
Suite 670
Chicago, IL 60631
312/714-8880
312/714-8886 fax

National Committee for Quality Assurance (NCQA)
1350 New York Avenue, NE
Suite 700
Washington, DC 20005
202/628-5788
202/628-0344 fax

Utilization Review Accreditation Commission (URAC)
1130 Connecticut Avenue, NW,
Suite 450
Washington, DC 20036
202/296-0120
202/296-0690

APPENDIX 4
STATE HEALTH INSURANCE AUTHORITIES

ALABAMA
Insurance Commissioner
P.O. Box 303351
Montgomery, AL 36120-3351
334/269-3550

ALASKA
Director of Insurance
State Office Building, 9th Floor
333 Willoughby
Juneau, AK 99801
907/465-2515

ARIZONA
Director of Insurance
2910 N. 44th Street, Suite 210
Phoenix, AZ 85018
602/912-8420

ARKANSAS
Insurance Commissioner
1123 S. University Avenue,
  Suite 400
Little Rock, AR 72204
501/686-2900

CALIFORNIA
Insurance Commissioner
300 Capitol Mall, Suite 100
Sacramento, CA 95814
916/445-5544

COLORADO
Insurance Commissioner
1560 Broadway, Suite 850
Denver, CO 80202
303/894-7499

CONNECTICUT
Insurance Commissioner
P. O. Box 816
Hartford, CT 06142-0816
203/297-3802

DELAWARE
Insurance Commissioner
148 Silver Lake Blvd.
P.O. Box 7007
Dover, DE 19903
302/739-4251

DISTRICT OF COLUMBIA
Superintendent of Insurance
441 4th Street, NW
Washington, DC 20001
202/727-8000

FLORIDA
Insurance Commissioner
200 Gaines Street
Tallahassee, FL 32399-0300
904/922-3100

GEORGIA
Insurance Commissioner
716 W. Cower
2 Martin Luther King Jr. Drive
Atlanta GA 30334
404/656-2056

HAWAII
Insurance Commissioner
250 S. King Street, 5th Floor
Honolulu, HI 96813
808/586-2799

IDAHO
Insurance Commissioner
P.O. Box 83720
Boise, Idaho 83720-0043
208/334-2250

ILLINOIS
Director of Insurance
320 W. Washington St.
Springfield, IL 62767
217/782-4515

INDIANA
Insurance Commissioner
311 W. Washington Street,
  Suite 300
Indianapolis, IN 46204
317/232-2385

IOWA
Insurance Commissioner
Lucas Building
Des Moines, IA 50319
515/281-5705

KANSAS
Insurance Commissioner
420 SW 9th Street
Topeka, KS 66612
502/564-3630

KENTUCKY
Insurance Commissioner
P.O. Box 517
Frankfort, KY 40602
502/564-3630

LOUISIANA
Insurance Commissioner
P. O. Box 94214
Baton Rouge, LA 70804-9214
504-342-5900

MAINE
Superintendent of Insurance
34 State House Station
Augusta, ME 04333
207/624-8475

MARYLAND
Insurance Commissioner
501 St. Paul Place
Baltimore, MD 21202
410/333-6300

MASSACHUSETTS
Insurance Commissioner
470 Atlantic Avenue
Boston, MA 02210-2223
617/521-7794

MICHIGAN
Insurance Commissioner
P. O. Box 30220
Lansing, MI 48909-7720
517/373-9273

MINNESOTA
Insurance Commissioner
133 E. 7th Street
St. Paul, MN 55101
612/269-6848

MISSISSIPPI
Insurance Commissioner
P.O. Box 79
Jackson, MS 39205
601/359-3569

MISSOURI
Director of Insurance
301 W. High Street,
  Room 630
Jefferson City, MO 65101
314/751-4126

MONTANA
Insurance Commissioner
P. O. Box 4009
Helena, MT 59604-4009
406/444-2040

NEBRASKA
Director of Insurance
941 O Street, Suite 400
Lincoln, NE 68508
602/471-2201

NEVADA
Insurance Commissioner
1665 Hot Springs Road,
#152
Carson City, NV 8710
702/687-4270

NEW HAMPSHIRE
Insurance Commissioner
169 Manchester St.
Concord, NH 03301-5151
603/271-2261

NEW JERSEY
Insurance Commissioner
20 W. State Street, CN325
Trenton, NJ 08625
609/292-5360

NEW MEXICO
Superintendent of Insurance
P. O. Drawer 1269
Santa Fe, NM 87504
505/827-4500

NEW YORK
Superintendent of Insurance
160 W. Broadway
New York, NY 10013
212/602-0492

NORTH CAROLINA
Insurance Commissioner
P. O. Box 26387
Raleigh, NC 27611
919/733-7349

NORTH DAKOTA
Insurance Commissioner
600 E. Boulevard, 5th Floor
State Capitol
Bismark, ND 58505-0320
701/328-2440

OHIO
Director of Insurance
2100 Stella Court
Columbus, OH 43215-1067
614/644-2651

OKLAHOMA
Insurance Commissioner
P. O. Box 53408
Oklahoma City, OK 73152-3408
405/521-2828

OREGON
Insurance Commissioner
350 Winter Street NE
Salem, OR 97310
503/378-4271

PENNSYLVANIA
Insurance Commissioner
1326 Strawberry Square
Harrisburg, PA 17128
717/787-5173

RHODE ISLAND
Insurance Commissioner
233 Richmond Street, Suite 233
Providence, RI 02903-4233
401/277-2223

SOUTH CAROLINA
Insurance Commissioner
P. O. Box 10015
Columbia, SC 29202-3105
803/737-6117

SOUTH DAKOTA
Director of Insurance
500 East Capitol
Pierre, SD 57501-5070
605-773-3563

TENNESSEE
Insurance Commissioner
500 James Robertson Parkway,
5th Floor
Nashville, TN 37243
615/741-6464

TEXAS
Insurance Commissioner
P. O. Box 149104
Austin, TX 78714-9104
512/463-6464

UTAH
Insurance Commissioner
State Office Building, #3110
Salt Lake City, UT 84114
801/538-3800

VERMONT
Insurance Commissioner
89 Main Street, Drawer 20
Montpelier, VT 05620-3101

VIRGINIA
P. O. Box 1157
Richmond, VA 23218
804/371-9741

WASHINGTON
Insurance Commissioner
P. O. Box 40255
Olympia, WA 98504-0255
360/753-7301

WEST VIRGINIA
Insurance Commissioner
P. O. Box 50540
Charleston, WV 25305
304/558-3386

WISCONSIN
Insurance Commissioner
P. O. Box 7873
Madison, WI 53707-7873
608/266-0102

WYOMING
Insurance Commissioner
Herschler Building, 3E
122 W. 25th Street
Cheyenne, WY 82002
307/777-7401

MAJOR U.S. HEALTH INSURANCE COMPANIES

Aetna Life Insurance Company
151 Farmington Ave.
Hartford, CT 06156
203/273-0123
203/273-6348 fax

**American Family Life
Insurance Company
of Columbus**
1923 Wynnton Rd.
Columbus, GA 31999
706/323-3431
706/596-3596 fax

**American Lincoln Insurance
Company**
One Alico Plaza
Wilmington, DE
302/594-2000
302/428-6019 fax

**AMEX Life Assurance
Company**
1650 Los Gamos Dr.
San Rafael CA 94903-1899
415/492-7000
415/492-7570

**American Medical Security
Insurance Company**
3100 AMS Blvd.
Green Bay, WI 54313
414/431-1111
414/431-2222

**Arkansas Blue Cross and
Blue Shield**
601 Gaines
Little Rock, AR 72201
501/378-2000
501/378-3258 fax

**Bankers Life and
Casualty Company**
222 Merchandise
Mart Plaza
Chicago, IL 60654-2001
312/396-6000
312/396-5900 fax

**Blue Cross Blue Shield
of Connecticut**
370 Bassett Rd.
North Haven, CT 06473
203/239-8454

**Blue Cross Blue Shield
of Florida**
533 Riverside Ave.
Jackson, FL 32202
904/791-6111

**Blue Cross Blue Shield
of Kansas**
1133 SW Topeka Blvd.
Topeka, KS 66629
913/291-7000

**The Colonial Life Insurance
Company of America**
8 Sylvan Way
Parsippany, NJ 07054-0216
201/631-2000
201/455-0189 fax

Colonial Life and Accident Insurance Company
1200 Colonial Life Blvd.
Columbia, SC 299210
803/798-7000
803/772-0251 fax

Continental Assurance Company
CNA Plaza
Chicago, IL 60685
312/822/5000
312/822-6419 fax

Connecticut General Life Insurance Company
900 Cottage Grove Rd.
Bloomfield, CT 06002
203/726-6000

CUNA Mutual Insurance Society
5910 Mineral Point Rd.
Madison, WI 53705
608/238-5851
608/238-0830 fax

Combined Insurance Company of America
123 Walker Dr.
Chicago, IL 60606
312/701-3000
312/701-3701 fax

Employers Health Insurance Company
1100 Employers Blvd.
De Pere, WI 54115
414/336-1100
414/336-2338 fax

Fortis Benefits Insurance Company
500 Bielenberg Dr.
Woodbury, MN 55125
612/738-4000
612/738-5356 fax

Golden Rule Insurance Company
712 Eleventh St.
Lawrenceville, IL 62439
618/943-8000
618/943-8031 fax

Great-West Life and Annuity Insurance Company
8515 E. Orchard Rd.
Englewood, CO 80111
303/689-3000
303/689-4321 fax

Hartford Life and Accident Insurance Company
200 Hopmeadow St.
Simsbury, CT 06070
203/843-8291
203/843-3057 fax

Health care Services Corporation
233 N. Michigan Ave.
Chicago, IL 60601
312/938-6680
312/861-0226 fax

Home Life Financial Assurance Company
221 E. Fourth St.
Cincinnati, OH 45202-4151
909/980-4000

IHSD Health Services Corp.
636 Grand Ave.
Des Moines, IA 50309
515/245-4500

Life Insurance Company of North America
1601 Chestnut St.
2 Liberty Place
Philadelphia, PA 19192-2235
215/761-1000
215/761-5606 fax

Jefferson-Pilot Life Insurance Company
100 N. Greene St.
Greensboro, NC 27401
910/691-3000
910/691-3938 fax

John Alden Life Insurance Company
5100 Gamble Dr.
St. Louis Park, MN 55416
3105/715-3100
305/715-3815 fax

John Hancock Mutual Life Insurance Company
John Hancock Plaza
Boston, MA 02117
617/572-6000
617/572-1799 fax

Massachusetts Mutual Life Insurance Company
1295 State St.
Springfield, MA 01111
413/788-8411
413/744-6038 fax

Metropolitan Life Insurance Company
One Madison Avenue, Area 9H
New York, NY 10010-3690
212/578-2211
212/578-7298 fax

Mutual of Omaha Insurance Company
Mutual of Omaha Plaza
Omaha, NE 68172
402/342-7600
402/351-2775 fax

New York Life Insurance Company
51 Madison Ave.
New York, NY 10010
212/576-7000
212/447-4156 fax

The Northwest Mutual Life Insurance Company
720 E. Wisconsin Ave.
Milwaukee, MI 53202
414/471-1444
414/299-2021 fax

The Paul Revere Life Insurance Company
18 Chestnut St.
Worcester, MA 01608-1528
508/799-4441
508/831-3488 fax

Physicians Mutual Insurance Company
2600 Dodge
Omaha, NE 68131
402/633-1000
402/633-6096 fax

PM Group Life Insurance Company
100 W. Clarendon, Suite 2000
Phoenix, AZ 85103
714/640-3011
714/760-4829 fax

Principal Mutual Life Insurance Company
711 High Street
Des Moines, IA 50392-0120
515/247-5111
515/247-5930 fax

Provident Life and Accident Insurance Company
One Fountain Square
Chattanooga, TN 37402
615/755-1011
615/755-7224 fax

The Prudential Insurance Company of America
Prudential Plaza
Newark, NJ 07102-2992
201/802-6000
201/802-8906 fax

Standard Insurance Company
1100 SW Sixth Ave.
Portland, OR 97204
503/325-7000
503/321-7935 fax

Time Insurance Company
501 W. Michigan Avenue
Milwaukee, MI 53201
414/271-3011
414/244-0472 fax

The Travelers Insurance Company
One Tower Square
Hartford, CT 06183
203/277-0111

Trustmark Life Insurance Company
400 Field Drive
Lake Forest, IL 60045-2581
708/615-1500
708/615-3910 fax

Union Fidelity Life Insurance Company
5050 N. Broadway
Chicago, IL 60640
312/701-3700
312/701-3701 fax

United American Insurance Company
2909 N. Buckner Blvd.
Dallas, TX 75228
214/328-2841

The United States Insurance Company
125 Maiden Lane
New York, NY 10038
212/709-6000
212/709-8707 fax

UNUM Life Insurance Company of America
2211 Congress St.
Portland, ME 04122
207/770-2211
207/770-9205 fax

Washington National Life Insurance Company of America
214 Jefferson St.
Lafayette, LA 70501
318/233-0230
318/237-2652 fax

APPENDIX 6
MAJOR U.S. MANAGED CARE COMPANIES

Aetna Health Plans
1000 Middle Street
Middletown, CT 06457
203/273-0123

Anthem Health Systems
5451 W. Lakeview Parkway,
South Dr.
Indianapolis, IN 46268
317/290-5600
317/298-6669 fax

Blue Cross Blue Shield Association
676 N. St. Clair St.
Chicago, IL 60611
312/440-6000

CIGNA Corporation
Hartford CT 06152
203/726-6000

CNA Managed Care
CNA Plaza, 27 South
Chicago, IL 60685
312/822-5000
312/822-1454

Community Care Network, Inc.
5251 Viewridge Ct.
San Diego, CA 92123
800/247-2898
619-278-1262 fax

Community Health Plan
1202 Troy-Schenectady Rd.
Latham, NY 12110
518/783-1864

Cost Care Physician Managed Network
660 Newport Center Dr., Suite 600
Newport Beach, CA 92660
714/729-4500
714/729-4650 fax

ETHIX Corporation
12655 SW Center St., Suite 540
Beaverton, OR 97005
503/643-8449

FHP, Inc.
9900 Talbert Ave.
Fountain Valley, CA 92708
714/963-7233

Focus Healthcare Management
7101 Executive Center Dr., Suite 375
Brentwood, TN 37027
615/377-9936

Health Economics Corporation
1300 W. Mockingbird
Dallas, TX 75247
214/905-4421
214-905-4427 fax

Healthsource
54 Regional Dr.
Concord, NH 03301
603/225-5077

Humana Health Care Plans
400 W. Main Street
Louisville, KY 40201
502/580-1000

Kaiser Foundaton Health Plan
Ordway Building
One Kaiser Plaza
Oakland, CA 94612
510/271-5910

Maxicare Health Plans
1149 Broadway
Los Angeles, CA 90015
213/742-0900

Medview Services
32991 Hamilton Ct.
Farmington Hills, MI 48334
313/448-5260
313/448-5262

MetLife HealthCare Network
57 Greens Farm Rd.
Westport, CT 06880
203/454-6100

PacifiCare Health Systems
5995 Plaza Dr.
Cypress, CA 90630
714/952-1121

Physician Corporation of
America
P. O. Box 025568
Miami, FL 33102
305/267-6633

Principal Health Care
1801 Rockville Pike, Suite 601
Rockville, MD 20852
301/881-1033
301/231-0020

Private Healthcare
Systems, Inc.
20 Maguire Rd.
Lexington, MA 02173
617/861-5500
617/862-3458

Prudential Insurance
56 N. Livingston Ave.
Roseland, NJ 07068
201/716-8000

QualMed
P. O. Box 1986
Pueblo, CO 81002-1986
719/542-0500

Sanus Corporation
1 Parker Plaza
400 Kelby St.
Fort Lee, NJ 07024
201/947-6000

State Mutual Life
Assurance Co.
440 Lincoln St.
Worcester, MA 01605
508/855-3278
508/885-2877

TakeCare
2300 Clayton Rd.
Cocord, CA 94520-2100
510/246-1300

Travelers Managed Care
Systems
1 Tower Plaza
Hartford, CT 06183-9083
203/954-2941

U.S. Healthcare
980 Jolly Rd.
Blue Bell, PA 19422-0770
215/628-4800
215/628-6858 fax

United HealthCare Corporation
P. O. Box 1459
Minneapolis, MN 55440-1459
612/936-1300

For more information about health maintenance organizations, contact:

American Association of Health Plans
1129 20th St. NW, Suite 600
Washington, DC 20036
202/778-3200
202/331-7487 fax

APPENDIX 7
MAJOR U.S. THIRD-PARTY ADMINISTRATORS

Accordia National
P.O. Box 1551
Charlestown, WV 25326
304/374-0737

Accordia, Inc.
120 Monument Circle
Indianapolis, IN 46204
606/223-0331

**American Medical
Security, Inc.**
P.O. Box 19032
Green Bay, WI 54307-9032
800/232-5432

**Associated Third Party
Administrators**
1999 Harrison Street,
Suite 500
Oakland, CA 94612
510/451-8564

CENTRA Benefit Services
1255 W. 15th Street,
Suite 1000
Plano, TX 75075
214/516-2600

CoreSource
630 Dundee Rd,
Suite 340
Northbrook, IL 60062
708/559-2420

Corporate Healthcare Financing
111 S. Calvert Street, Suite 2670
Baltimore, MD 21202
410/837-2580

EBP Health Plans, Inc.
435 Ford Rd., #500
Minneapolis, MN 55426
612/546-4353

**Executive Risk
Consultants, Inc.**
P.O. Box 166007
Altamonte Springs, FL 32716
407/788-1717

First Health
6975 Union Park Center, Suite 600
Midvale, UT 84047
801/568-5500

Frank Gates Service Company
P.O. Box 16580
Columbus, OH 43216-6580
614/793-8000

Godwins, Brooke & Dickerson
P. O. Box 66
Winston-Salem, NC 27102-0066
910/748-1120

R.E. Harrington, Inc.
55 E. Jackson Blvd.,
8th Floor
Chicago, IL 60604
312/346-2626

HealthPlan Services
525 Central Park, Building #1,
Suite 400
Oklahoma City, OK 73105
405/521-0082

**Lipman Insurance
Administrators, Inc.**
39420 Liberty Street, Suite 260
Fremont, CA 94538
510/796-4676

Managed Care of America
820 Parish Street
Pittsburgh, PA 15220
412/922-2803

Zenith Administrators
7645 Metro Blvd.
Minneapolis, MN 55435
612/835-7035

For more information about third-party administrators, contact:

Society of Professional Benefit Administrators
2 Wisconsin Circle, Suite 670
Chevy Chase, MD 20815-7003
301/718-7722
301/718-9440 FAX

APPENDIX 8
HEALTH CARE RESOURCES ON THE WORLD WIDE WEB

American Academy of Allergy, Asthma and Immunology
http://execpc.com/ ~ edi/aaaai.html

American Academy of Child and Adolescent Psychiatry
http://www.med.umich.edu/aacap/homepage.html

American Academy of Dermatology
http://www.derm-info.com/EPA

American Academy of Emergency Medicine
http://www.trail.com/ ~ aaem/index.html

American Academy of Orthopaedic Surgeons
http://www.aaos.org

American Academy of Pain Management
http://www.sonnet.com/aapm

American Academy of Pediatrics
http://www.aap.org

American Association of Health Plans
http://www.aahp.org

American Association for Medical Transcription
http://www.aamt.org.aamt

American Chiropractic Association
http://www.cais.net/acn

American College of Cardiology
http://www.acc.org

American Dental Association
http://www.ada.org

American Diabetes Association
http://www.diabetes.org

American Health Information Management Association
http://www.ahima.org

American Heart Association
http://www.amhrt.org

American Medical Association
http://www.ama-assn.org

American Medical Specialty Organization
http://www.amso.com

American Medical Student Association
http://med-amsa.bu.edu/AMSA/AMSA.hml

American Physical Therapy Association
http://www.netspot.unisa.edu.au/pt

American Podiatric Medical Association
http://www.apma.org

American Psychological Association
http://www.apa.org

American Red Cross
http://www.crossnet.org

Avicenna
http://www.avicenna.com

Centers for Disease Control and Prevention
http://www.cdc.org

Community Health Management Information Systems Resource Center
http://www.chmis.org

Food and Drug Administration
http://www.fda.gov/fdahomepage.html

Galaxy Medicine
http://galaxy.einet.net/galaxy/Medicine.html

GNN Health and Medicine
http://www.nearnet.gnn.com/wic/med.toc.html

Health Administration Resources
http://www.mercer.peachnet.edu/www/health/health.html

Health Care Facilities Institute
http://www.hfi.org

Healthcare Financial Management Association
http://www.hfma.org

Health Care Financing Administration
http://www.hcfa.gov

Health Information and Management Systems Society
http://www.himss.org

Health Resources and Services Administration
http://www.os.dhhs.gov/hrsa

HospitalWeb
http://neuro-www.mgh.harvard.edu/hospitalweb.hclk

Indian Health Service
http://www.tucson.ihs.gov

International Committee of the Red Cross
http://www.icrc.ch

International Society for Technology Assessment in Health Care
http://www.neomed.com

Integrated Healthcare Association
http://www.ihc.org

Internet Health Resources
http://www.ihr.com

Medical EquipNet
http://www.solumed.com

Medical Matrix
http://www.slackinc.com/matrix

Medical Records Institute
http://www.medrecinst.com

Medlinks
http://www.medlinks.com/links.htm

Medscape
http://www.medscape.com

MedSearch
http://www.medsearch.com

Morbidity and Mortality Weekly Report
http://www.cdc.gov/epo/mmwr/mmwr.html

Multimedia Medical Reference Library
http://www.tiac.net/users/jtward/images.html

National Committee for Quality Assurance
http://www.ncqa.org

National Institutes of Health
http://www.nih.gov

National Cancer Institute
http://www.nci.gov

National Eye Institute
http://www.nei.gov

National Heart, Lung and Blood Institute
http://www.nhlbi.nih.gov/nhlbi.html

National Institute of Allergy and Infectious Disease
http://www.niaid.nih.gov

National Institute on Alcohol Abuse and Alcoholism
http://www.niaaa.nih.gov

National Institute of Arthritis and Musculoskeletal and Skin Disorders
http://www.nih.gov.niams

National Institute of Child Health and Human Development
http://www.nih.gov/nichd

National Institute of Dental Research
http://www.nidr.nig.gov

National Institute of Diabetes and Digestive and Kidney Diseases
http://www.niddk.nih.gov

National Institute on Drug Abuse
http://www.nida.gov

National Institute of Environmental Health Sciences
http://www.niehs.gov

National Institute of General Medical Sciences
http://www.nih.gov/nigms

National Institute of Mental Health
http://www.nimh.nih.gov

National Institute of Neurological Disorders and Stroke
http://www.nih.gov/nids

National Institute of Nursing Research
http://www.nih.gov/ninr

National Center for Human Genome Research
http://www.nchgr.nig.gov

National Center for Research
http://www.ncrr.nih.gov

National Organization of Rare Diseases
http://www.w2.com/nordl.htm

National Science Foundation
http://stis.nsf.gov

Occupational Safety and Health Administration
http://www.osha.gov

PharmWeb
http://www.mcc.ac.uk/pharmacy

Physician's GenRx Online
http://www.genrx.com

Physician's Guide to the Internet
http://saturn.netrep.com/home/pgi

Physicians Online
http://www.po.com/hyper.html

Radiological Society of North America
http://www.rsna.org

Society of Critical Care Medicine
http://execpc.com/sccm

U.S. Department of Health and Human Services
http://www.os.dhhs.gov

U.S. Public Health Service
http://phs.oh.dhhs.gov/phs/phs.html

The Virtual Hospital
http://indy.radiology.uiowa.edu/VirtualHospital.html

Yahoo Health
http://www.yahoo.com/health

World Health Organization
http://www.who.ch

WWW Virtual Library: Medicine
http://www.ohsu.edu/cliniweb/wwwvl